BRUCE

Dorothy L. Wegman
1979

BRUCE

by Dorothy Wyman

Southern Publishing Association, Nashville, Tennessee

Copyright © 1979 by
Southern Publishing Association

This book was
Edited by Gerald Wheeler
Designed by Mark O'Connor
Cover photo by Mark O'Connor

Type set: 10/12 Melior

Printed in U.S.A.

Library of Congress Cataloging in Publication Data

Wyman, Dorothy, 1918-
  Bruce.

  1. Friedreich's ataxia—Biography. 2. Wyman, Bruce,
1944-
RC406.F7W95   362.4'3'0926   [B]   78-23504
ISBN   0-8127-0217-4

Chapter 1

The worn wheelchair creaked and protested as my husband labored to maneuver it up the church steps. I flung my purse over my left arm, ran up the stairs ahead of him, and tugged at the heavy door. It gave way suddenly, and a smiling, portly man pushed it open wide.

"Can I help you, sir?" he asked.

Lynn placed his booted foot against the lift bar and eased the front wheels of the chair to the concrete floor of the entryway. "Thank you, but I can manage just fine."

"Yes, I suppose you can." The elderly man placed his gnarled hand on my husband's arm in a kindly gesture. "You've had lots of practice, I expect." Still holding the door open with his body, he leaned forward and grasped the hand of the stooped figure in the wheelchair. "Bruce, we are so happy to have you here this morning!" His deep voice rang with genuine pleasure.

My son made a real effort to sit straight in his chair. Deep brown eyes sparkled, and a wide, pleasant smile spread over his angular face. His dark hair, cropped short in a crew cut, glistened in the morning sun. "Thank you, Art," Bruce said. "I'm glad to be here, too."

The words came clear and distinct, not an easy feat for the misshapen young man whose useless legs fell to one side as the wheelchair bumped a small floor latch in the doorway. My husband grasped him under the arms and straightened his body into a more comfortable position. I bent over and fastened each leg in an improvised seat belt that enabled him to sit more securely and with reasonable safety.

"We've a place reserved for him at the very front of the church, Mr. Wyman."

I looked up to see the triumphant features of a handsome young man, younger yet than my son, but nevertheless a minister.

"Hello, Tony, we made it!" I greeted him.

The young minister smiled at me, and I thought I detected a mistiness in his dark eyes not usually there. He reminded me greatly of Bruce.

"I never doubted that you would, Mrs. Wyman. This has to be one of the happiest days of my ministry." He placed one hand heavily on Bruce's head and shook it from side to side in a brotherly sort of greeting. "Today is your big day, right, Bruce?"

"Right, Tony!"

The bond of loving friendship between the two young men was unmistakable.

My husband eased the wheelchair over the obstacle and followed Tony into the church. Deep purple carpeting impeded the wheels of the chair, and Lynn pushed hard against the handgrips. All heads in the congregation turned, and almost as one they spoke, "Good morning, Bruce. God bless you."

Bruce smiled and waved his weakened hands.

Down the aisle to the front of the church my husband rolled our son, stopping momentarily along the way as many hands reached out to clasp Bruce's. Lynn turned and backed the wheelchair into position, stooped and inquired in a whisper about Bruce's comfort, then joined me in the second pew. As I slid over to make room for him I felt a tap on my shoulder. When I turned I saw a stout woman, slightly graying, grinning broadly at me. Her colorful, floor-length print dress seemed to accentuate her size, yet it lent an air of cheerfulness about her. "We're so happy you could come and so glad to see Bruce," she whispered.

Her husband, without speaking, nodded his agreement. He wasn't a large man, and beside his wife he appeared diminutive. However pleasant his features, he smiled only with his eyes and offered me an open hymnal. I thanked him, acknowledged his wife's hospitality, and as I turned back to my husband the organ resounded with the opening notes of "What a Friend We Have in Jesus." At the pulpit the older resident minister said, "Shall we stand, please?"

The room bustled expectantly as the forty or fifty people in the congregation rose to their feet. As the words "What a Friend we have in Jesus, All our sins and griefs to bear" rang out on the morning air the young intern minister, Tony Finch, thoughtfully stepped down from the rostrum and, with an open songbook placed where Bruce could read, stood beside our son. His melodious voice, deep and vibrant, rose in exultation above the others. I felt a lump in my throat and for a moment listened to the chorus of happy voices. One could not mistake the anticipation they felt this particular Sabbath morning. On this April day, 1973, they had gathered to witness our Bruce's baptism into the Seventh-day Adventist faith.

I looked at Bruce. His deep-set eyes mirrored the joy I knew throbbed in his heart. After a long, exhausting search he had found his religious home, and he reveled in its faith, its security, and most of all its hope. His voice pealed forth in song, perhaps a little off-key but matching the exuberance in the voice of his minister friend. How sure of himself he seemed, confident in his chosen faith and rejoicing with his church family in its promises.

As the organ, pedal-soft and quiet, played another chorus I heard the minister say, "Let us pray." I stole a glance at Bruce. His head, never in complete control, dropped roughly to his chest. Bowing my own, I noticed Tony place his arm about Bruce's shoulders, his face etched in concern. I closed my eyes. As "Our Father, which art in heaven" reverberated through the church I felt my tense muscles relax. My memory slipped back across the years to a small Oregon lumber camp, where first I had noticed that my son did not respond normally to the usual activities of a three-year-old.

Bruce has been confined to a wheelchair since 1962. Of necessity he leads a quite limited life. But it has not always been so. Born Richard Bruce Wyman on April 13, 1944, he made his debut in Portland, Oregon, in the wee hours of a showery spring morning.

My husband, Lynn, and I, along with our two older children, Connie and David, had moved into a crowded wartime housing development in north Portland during the early months of World War II. Lynn worked as a welder leadman with a crew of fifteen or twenty welders under him at the Swan Island shipyard. Huge tankers slid down the ways here into the broad Willamette River at the rate of one every twelve days. In addition he worked a half shift at Hyster Company as a welder too. It was grilling, monotonous work, but because of a chronic duodenal ulcer, developed after the death of our first child, Dale, in a tragic accident, the armed forces had rejected his application. Patriotism flowed freely in those days, and the exhaustive routine was my husband's contribution to the war effort. We were more than glad to put up with the inconveniences of a crowded city built to accommodate many thousands less than were stuffed into its concrete jungles. Gas rationing, food stamps, waiting in long lines to buy our share of scarce commodities, cars with every possible commuter crammed inside, odd hours, and meals at midnight were a way of life.

It was on one such night that Lynn had barely begun his midnight luncheon when I suddenly went into severe labor. The due date was still a week or two away for our expected baby. But it hadn't learned to read calendars and insisted now was the appointed time. With little grace, my husband picked me up and ran to the car. He literally flung me into it and drove the thirteen miles to Wilcox Memorial Hospital with all the speed the 1937 vintage Nash could produce. Even refusing to stop for red lights failed to attract a law officer to guide us through traffic. I breathed a silent prayer that somehow we would make it safely and before the baby arrived. We did.

Less than an hour later I shook the cobwebs from my mind and tried to convince myself that the nurse standing over me was actually saying, "Wake up, Mrs. Wyman. You have a beautiful baby boy." My back twisted in tangled muscle spasms. I couldn't believe that with such excruciating pain I had already given birth. I must have complained.

"I'm sorry, Dorothy." From somewhere in the sterile expanse of the delivery room I heard my doctor's voice. "You've had a very fast and painful delivery, but it couldn't be avoided. The baby was in an extremely difficult position and required a lot of turning. That's why you're so miserable."

Groaning, I tried to raise up to see the bundle of new life cradled in the nurse's arms. My body refused, simply too tired to make the effort. The nurse laid the wriggling baby across my stomach and held him securely.

"Isn't he precious? Just look at that mop of black hair!"

The doctor chuckled. "Lynn's going to be proud of this one. He certainly shows his Indian ancestry!"

They were right. A darkskinned little creature with jet-black hair, his tiny face puckered and frowning, he searched for a chubby hand to stuff in a hungry mouth.

"See there, he's looking for the dining room already!" The doctor snapped paper-thin gloves off his large hands, and someone wheeled me toward my room.

Born with unusual stamina, Bruce survived a bout with whooping cough contracted at the age of two weeks that nearly overcame his three-year-old sister and two-year-old brother. Even though I was able to nurse him only two and a half months, he didn't complain when I offered him a bottle. He laughed and cooed, wriggled and squirmed, his way right into our hearts. Only his bath brought out the worst in him. Arms flailing, he protested loud and long from its beginning until he felt the security of his warm, soft clothing again. Perhaps it might have been the first of many indications that he was not completely normal. If so, it escaped me.

Bruce did all of the things one expects small babies to

do, and he did them well. Everyone remarked about how erect he sat at four months. He crept at an early age. His coordination seemed normal until he began to walk. Even then he did well as long as he grasped an object, but he refused to walk alone. We thought he just lacked confidence in himself.

In the meantime my husband continued shouldering the heavy work load, snatching what little time he could to enjoy his family. Such an exhausting routine I'm sure a lesser man could not have coped with. Eventually Lynn's body rebelled. His doctor insisted that he must change his pace and get away from the dense welding smoke that filled the double hulls of the ships. Pulling all the strings available to him and agreeing to go into another priority industry, Lynn managed to get out of the shipyards.

In June, 1945, we moved to the small logging and lumber community of Lorane, Oregon. My husband went to work in the Chambers Lumber Company mill, and we began a whole new way of life. At heart we were really country people, and neither of us had liked living in a large city.

Fourteen months old now, and with his usual avid curiosity, Bruce responded with fascination to every phase of the moving process. He loved spending a week with his Uncle Bert and Aunt Ellen while we tried to make some semblance of a home out of an old lumber camp shack. It was a challenge, but we enjoyed every moment of it. We were happy to have our family closer to nature and a simpler life.

I will never forget the first night in our new home. The out-of-doors captivated Connie and David, and they couldn't wait to explore their new world. Its boundaries must have seemed endless to their four- and two-and-a-half-year-old minds after the confinement of a small yard in a wartime housing project.

The house was still pretty cluttered and hectic. Tired of the constant attention of adoring cousins, Bruce was cross and irritable. Lynn carried him into the house, and I cleared a place for him on the sofa. The expression on his face amazed us. After everything being strange and unfamiliar around him, at last he had found something he recognized. His black eyes sparkled, and his lips crinkled into that charming smile so much a part of him. Curious hands explored the upholstery. He squealed with delight and began bouncing against the back of the sofa. In less than five minutes he fell asleep.

Once settled in our mountain home, the children and I enjoyed a lazy summer. Our fifth child well on the way, I treasured the slower pace we lived. Leisurely walks beneath the stately Douglas fir forest that surrounded our place, afternoons with a book while I rested on a carpet of maidenhair fern and watched the children play, seemed like moments out of a pleasant dream.

August came, and the Japanese surrendered. The horrors of the war in the Pacific, the A-bomb, Hiroshima and Nagasaki, were over. As our family stood in the yard waving at some neighbors who drove by, honking their car horn wildly in celebration of a long war's end, I stood Bruce on the lawn and walked away from him.

"Look, look." I grasped my husband's arm. "He's standing alone!" For weeks we had tried over and over again to persuade him to walk, but he refused even to stand alone. Now, in the excitement of the moment, he stood unaided, both arms waving as he mimicked Connie and David.

Lynn squatted a few feet from him and held out his hands. "Hey, fella, come see me!"

Bruce reached for his daddy and almost took a step, but instead plopped his chubby self on the ground. Again and again I stood him on his feet, but no amount of coaxing encouraged him to walk. He would stand alone, but he would not take a step. Finally we gave it up and all returned to the house and a supper grown cold in the excitement of surrender and one little boy, who had learned at sixteen months that feet were made for standing on.

The new baby arrived prematurely in September. We christened her Nova Lynne. Bruce adored her.

In an era of wringer washing machines and outdoor clotheslines, even the indoors became a bit soggy during a rainy Oregon winter. Clothes racks were permanent pieces of furniture. One evening as we all sat about the living room I asked Connie to bring me a diaper from the clothes rack that stood in its perpetual place by the wood heater. Always a miniature mother, she walked her little brother across the room.

"Here, Dicky Bruce," she smiled as she spoke her favorite name for him. "Would you like to help? Take the diaper to Mommy." Without realizing he held nothing more than a flimsy piece of cloth in his hands, he walked the full length of the room and deposited the diaper on my lap. Connie stared in disbelief. David jumped up and down.

"Daddy! Look, Daddy, look! Brucie can walk!"

Lynn dropped his evening paper. "Well, I'll be switched!" He grabbed him up and hugged him close. "See, I knew you could do it. Let me see you walk to Connie."

His sister held out her hands. A little ham at heart, Bruce was ready to perform. Back and forth between various members of the family he marched until his legs would no longer hold him up. He bubbled over with happiness. While he hadn't broken any records—that was for sure—to our little family nestled in a cozy old shack, a baby boy finally walking alone at eighteen months was a real achievement.

As the children grew older they became quite fond of our lumber camp home. It never seemed to occur to them that bare fir-board walls were unusual. Lack of indoor plumbing simply made for adventure as they journeyed back and forth to the outside privy. Even baths in a round galvanized laundry tub were fun times. But it was the washtub that gave me my first hint that Bruce had a physical problem.

"Straighten out your legs, Brucie," I said as I lathered a washcloth, "so I can scrub you clean. You're a dirty little boy!"

"No, Mommy, it hurts!"

"What hurts?"

"My legs. They always hurt when you baff me!"

"Oh, come on, now. It doesn't hurt to get clean."

I moved him over in the crowded tub to make room to straighten his legs and pulled on them gently. They seemed tense and resistive.

"No, Mommy, please, it hurts!"

At three-and-a-half Bruce still disliked bathing and often conjured up excuses to get out of various things he didn't like doing. To assure myself now was not one of those times, I examined him carefully for bruises, scratches, or slivers. I found nothing.

"Come look at Bruce's legs, would you, please?"

My husband reluctantly eased himself out of his comfortable chair and knelt by the tub. "What's the matter? Did you fall and bruise your leg or something, fella?"

"Nope."

Lynn pulled on his legs. Pain registered on Bruce's sun-tanned face, but he didn't complain. "Oh, I think he's just got a cramp. I get 'em, too, when I get crammed into this tub!" He smeared a cluster of soap bubbles on Bruce's nose and went back to his book. "You mothers are all alike. Gotta find something to worry about."

I finished his bath, but as I filled and emptied the tub twice more for Connie's and David's baths I could not forget the pained look on Bruce's face whenever I applied any pressure against his knees. Even after I had tucked the children in their beds and had listened to three childish prayers, I couldn't erase from my mind the subtle anxiety, the growing fear, that something was not right. We had lost one son, and I couldn't bear the thought of losing another, or even having anything seriously wrong with my babies.

The summer months found the children busily exploring the lush forest surrounding our home. Bruce, always eager for new adventures, followed Connie and David everywhere. Quite often they played at an abandoned old cabin several hundred yards from the house. The forest, cool and inviting, completely encircled the small meadow where the cabin sat, and sometimes they played there for hours at a time. A fallen fir, downed by some freakish storm, provided an improvised seesaw that Connie and David delighted in bouncing to its greatest heights. Bruce seemed to prefer quiet games and seldom attempted to play on the tree unless his sister and brother were otherwise occupied. His fear of falling was much more pronounced than theirs. He wanted to teeter only a little and abandoned it as soon as he thought one of the children might jump on the branches and swing him high. When they came home, David always arrived ahead of Connie and Bruce. If I asked why he hadn't waited for them, he would say, "Ah, Mom, Brucie is so slow, and he falls down so much. They're comin'." Connie, patient and considerate, never deserted him.

One evening as Lynn and I watched them arrive home, their feet making little dust puffs in the powder-fine dirt of the logging road, Bruce stumbled and fell. Connie stopped to help him up. Dust fairly flew as she slapped and brushed at his dirty T-shirt and pants. She fanned her hands through his ash-blond hair—hair that at birth had been so black—and made grimy smears down both sides of his prominent nose as she wiped the soil from around his tearful brown eyes.

"Lynn, do you think Bruce's knees look just right when he walks?" I asked. "It seems to me that he falls so much more than the other two did at his age."

My husband shaded his eyes against the setting sun and watched for a moment as the boy plodded up the road, his head craned to one side, eyes squinted, watching an early nighthawk catch his evening meal.

"Well, he does seem a little knock-kneed, but so what? I'm bowlegged. And look at him, he's not paying one bit of attention to where he's stepping. He's too interested in everything going on around him. There's no wonder he falls all the time."

"I suppose you're right. I'll have to admit he's full of curiosity. It doesn't take much to spark his imagination." The nighthawk swooped low. "He's probably wondering right now what it would be like to fly."

"Yeah," Lynn chuckled, "or wondering what a bug tastes like."

A peculiar odor from the kitchen, smelling much like scorched potatoes, cut our conversation short. Dashing inside, I once again pushed from my mind what must surely have been a clue to our son's physical condition.

We were happy that during the summer the telephone company had installed a shiny black phone in our living room, for winter came on strong that year. Sometime in January an unusual storm blew in that piled up thirty-seven inches of snow in the valley. The tall Douglas firs drooped with the heavy snow, and every shrub and fence carried a blob of white frosting. The beauty was breathtaking, but I had little time to enjoy it. Feverish and delirious, Bruce tossed on his cot in the children's bedroom. For some time recurring attacks of tonsillitis had plagued him, but this bout proved more serious than any previous ones. His temperature soared to 106.5 degrees. Electric lines had succumbed to the weight of the snow, and we were without power. Fortunately the telephone lines remained intact, for we were snowbound.

When snow falls west of the Cascades, it is wet and heavy, like soggy cement. Few vehicles can negotiate it. Getting Bruce to a doctor was out of the question. I called our family physician, Dr. Axley, in Cottage Grove and explained our predicament. With the telephone lines already crackling and threatening to break, he gave me explicit directions for emergency care, cautioning me of the severity of possible brain damage from an excessively high fever.

Luckily our medicine shelf held the necessary items. My husband and I began a constant battle to lower his temperature. Bruce lay limp and still, his dark skin flushed and burning. Frequent dips into tepid water—drying him only enough to keep him from dripping—and sponging with alcohol brought little protest from him. An occasional weak, "Please don't, Mommy," came whispered through dry, parched lips. Lacking ice that we could not produce without power, we improvised an ice bag, using snow, for his head. Unable to contact Dr. Axley again—for only minutes after his instructions, the telephone lines lay hidden in the deep snow—we prayed. Finally, thirty-six hours later, in the wee hours of the night, the fever broke. Once again his skin felt moist. His unruly hair made odd little patterns against his forehead as sweat beaded his brow. The short gasps for air gave way to deep breathing, and sound sleep overtook his exhausted body. Tired and spent, Lynn and I breathed a grateful prayer and tumbled into bed to rest the few remaining hours before dawn.

The next day my brother and his wife, in an old Model T Ford pickup, broke their way through the valley to our place. Those old cars, built high off the ground, had their compensations. Loaded with groceries they thought we might need, Bert and his wife were a welcome sight. However, the crisis with Bruce's illness over, we were not in any real bind. But we were grateful for their thoughtfulness. They crawled back into the old Model T, refusing our invitation to spend the night.

"Thank you, but we'd better not," Bert said as he revved up the noisy motor. "There may be others that need our aid." Of course he was right, for in an area where snow seldom presented a problem, highway crews had little time for an out-of-the-way lumber community.

Clear skies brought extremely cold weather, and the millpond froze solid, something the old-timers could not remember happening for many years. Without electric power for fifteen days, the local school closed. Teenagers gathered at our place by the dozens to play on the ice and frolic in the winter wonderland. Lynn, merely a boy grown taller and older, joined the fun. He dragged out long unused ice skates, and the air rang with laughter and shouts as he and the children glided and slid across the glassy pond. Although Bruce, as usual, recuperated quickly, he did not like the ice if left to maneuver on his own. Balancing on the slick surface seemed more than he could manage. We thought perhaps he still needed time to gain steadiness after his illness. Never adept at balance myself, Bruce and I toasted marshmallows over a fire, much to everyone's delight.

In another week or two warm weather returned. The snow and ice disappeared almost overnight, and everything settled back to a normal routine. Bruce was once again his cheerful self, playful and completely recovered. It seemed foolish to take a well boy to the doctor, and we didn't.

The remainder of the winter passed quickly. Connie was in school now. Every evening after the big yellow bus deposited her at our driveway, Bruce clamored for a school session, much to her pleasure. By the time spring fluttered in on its gossamer green wings, he had learned to print his name, knew some of the letters of the alphabet, and in squiggly figures made all the numbers.

But trying her best, she could not teach him to tie his shoelaces. He seemed to have five fingers and two thumbs on each hand. Although always a perfectionist, it was the first time we'd seen her become completely frustrated with him.

"Mamma, I can't do it. You've got to teach him to tie his shoelaces, or he'll be going to school with them all untied." I informed her we still had nearly two years before he would start school. Besides, tying shoestrings was the least of Bruce's worries. He just went on chewing on the neck of his T-shirt—a bad little habit we'd failed to break him of—and paid no attention to Connie's demands.

David and Bruce became real pals after Connie started school. When summer came he still tagged David about, emulating everything he did, even climbing a tall fir, which almost proved disastrous. A fall of thirty feet that momentarily knocked Bruce unconscious scared David and the rest of us nearly out of our wits. But it didn't produce any broken bones or serious cuts, and only a few nasty bruises. However, years later the fall did figure prominently in the search for Bruce's crippling handicap. But when it occurred it seemed only one more harrowing experience in the life of a growing family.

Bruce continued to have recurring attacks of tonsillitis, but never again as severe as the winter we'd been snowbound. During the summer of 1949 Dr. Axley concluded the tonsils would have to come out.

I still felt apprehensive about his clumsiness. Dr. Axley agreed that I had some reason for anxiety. "I'm sure it's only because of toxic substances in his body due to excessive tonsil infections," he told me one hot, muggy afternoon in his second-story office. "But we can't remove them now. Too much danger of polio during the heat of summer. Besides, he's had both measles and chicken pox in recent months. We'll give him time to build up some resistance. But I'm sure they'll have to come out before he goes to school."

"Will we have to take him to Eugene?" Cottage Grove had no hospital at that time.

"Oh, my, no. We'll do it right here in my office. I've forgotten how many tonsillectomies I've performed in that little room."

That fall my brother's daughter Nita came to live with us. Her parents had moved to Roseburg, Oregon, but she wanted to graduate with her class at Lorane High. So we pushed everything just a little closer in our crowded home and made room for her. We also made room for a new baby girl, Merrie Jo, born October 22, 1949. Nita had come to stay, with the agreement that she remain home from school for a week or so to mind the children while I took time out to have the baby. The arrangement worked perfectly. An honor student and an industrious young lady, Nita managed her schoolwork and our household with unbelievable skill. Her honey-blonde hair tied up in a scarf, bouncy curls escaping here and there, and blue eyes sparkling, she maneuvered our children with a brand of homespun psychology that often left us marveling at her teenage perception. The children adored her. They, especially Connie and Bruce, imitated her every move. Quickly she had gained the confidence of each one. In less time than we thought possible, Bruce could tie his shoelaces. She and her fiancé, Ken, actually enjoyed baby-sitting the children. I fear we often took advantage of their willingness. Rather than complaining, however, they insisted that Lynn and

I go out alone occasionally. The children always begged to stay with Nita and Ken, and we felt pampered.

As he had when Nova arrived, Bruce idolized his new baby sister. Together he and Nova would pull the kitchen table close to the big wood range, open the oven door for extra warmth, and we'd have a fun session giving Merrie Jo her bath. Although past four, Nova had to be watched closely. The baby's eyes fascinated her. Bruce took it upon himself to be Merrie Jo's protector.

"No, no, Nony!" He would grasp her exploring hands in his. "You mustn't poke her in the eyes. They're for lookin', not for pokin'."

In the spring of 1950 Lynn and his carloading partner accepted a new position in Cottage Grove. It involved the same type of work but offered a much better salary. Since our home belonged to the company Lynn worked for, we would now have to move. After a long search we found a place close to Lorane and not far from where we lived.

The big two-story log house seemed like a mansion to us after the crowded quarters in the old shack. An early settler's home, it too lacked a bathroom. But it did have a sink and cold water in a quaint old-fashioned kitchen. Four bedrooms—two upstairs and two down—would give all of us a chance to spread out. The boys chose one room upstairs and Connie the other. Nova and Baby Merrie would occupy a downstairs room. An expansive combination living and dining area took up nearly as much space as our whole lumber camp shack.

Our family was back to its original size now. Nita, after graduation, swore us to secrecy, and she and Ken eloped to Tacoma, Washington, where Ken's brother, a navy chaplain, married them. They made their home in a minisized apartment in Cottage Grove.

Dr. Axley decided the first week in June would be tonsillectomy time and set the date for a Monday morning. Ironically, we had made our moving arrangements for that weekend. Our many friends, without being called upon, rallied to our aid. The whole chore, complete with clean cupboards, dishes put away, and all the beds made up, took less than two days. Someone brought in a hot meal Sunday evening. With all the help and kind deeds bestowed upon us, I had Bruce bathed and snug in bed by 8 PM. His appointment with the doctor the next morning didn't seem to concern him a bit.

Before I retired, I slipped upstairs to check on the three eldest. All slept with exhausted contentment. In a heap on the floor by his bed, Bruce's pajamas lay in a tangled mess. From the time he had learned to dress himself, he had despised sleepwear. Although we always made him put them on, sometime during the night he shed them. This night I didn't bother to redress him, just pulled the blankets about him, planted a kiss on his forehead, and tiptoed out of the room.

When the alarm went off at 5 AM, I felt as if I had just crawled in bed. In my stomach it seemed that a thousand butterflies flitted about. However, Bruce bounced out of bed and dressed quickly, a rare occurrence indeed. To him it was all a big adventure. It continued to be so right up to the moment Mrs. Axley, the doctor's lovely wife and assistant, placed the ether mask over his face. Bruce's curiosity had sparked all sorts of questions about the surgical instruments and the procedure ahead of him.

"This is fun, Mom." He wrinkled his nose at me.

"I'm glad you're enjoying it, Bruce." *Oh, dear God, don't let him see how frightened I am.*

"Now breathe deep, Brucie." The nurse's instruction was his command. He did exactly as she told him.

"Can you count for me, Bruce?" Dr. Axley asked and pulled the last glove on his hand.

"One, two, three——four————five——" The numbers grew fainter and farther apart.

"That's good, Bruce. What comes after five?"

Instead of a spoken number, the most ominous sound I have ever heard rolled up from the deep recesses of his lungs.

O God, he's choking to death! Fear clutched me in a vicelike grip. Dr. Axley seemed unperturbed.

"He's perfectly all right. This is normal."

The sweet but nauseating odor of ether permeated the air, and I felt the room spin.

"Young lady, I think you need some fresh air. Go take a little walk, and be careful of those stairs."

Leaving Bruce made me feel guilty, but I knew the doctor was right. I stumbled out the door and clung to the railing as I eased myself down the stairs. When I reached the street my legs would hold me no longer. Sinking down on the last step, I buried my head between my knees.

"You're such a baby," I told myself. "Here you've had six children, and you can't even watch a tonsillectomy. You, who always wanted to be a nurse!" I hadn't reacted like this when we had Connie's tonsils removed, but that took place in a large modern hospital where the nurses had whisked her away to surgery. When she returned it was all over. Here I was a part of the whole scene. Scolding myself mentally, I walked a few yards down the street. Breathing deeply of the cool morning air, I felt much better. Back up the long flight of stairs I ran. *I'll see this through, or else!* But the door was locked.

"Dr. Axley?" My own voice sounded weak and ashamed.

"Oh, go get a cup of coffee or something and come back in about an hour. We haven't time to be picking you up off the floor!"

Although I felt guilty and frustrated, I secretly breathed a sigh of relief.

Back on the street the fragrance of bacon frying hung in the still air. Suddenly I remembered I hadn't had time for breakfast. I walked down the street to a restaurant and ordered a full meal. After the waitress sat a plate of steaming eggs, hashbrowns, and toast in front of me, I bowed my head in a moment of thanksgiving and prayer for the little boy who lay with his life in the hands of a kindly and competent physician.

"For thine is the kingdom, and the power, and the glory, for ever. Amen." The rustle of Sabbath School papers and hymnals, the sound of people being seated, brought me back from my memories. Bruce listened intently to something Tony whispered to him. From the young minister's gestures, I assumed that he was explaining the baptismal procedure. My son nodded and smiled and I lip-read the words, "OK, Tony."

After a few announcements and another hymn, the resident minister walked to the pulpit. "Dear friends," he said, "today is a momentous occasion for us. As you all know, the sermon will be short this morning, for we are going to witness the baptism of a very dear young man into our faith and the blessing of our heavenly Father."

I glanced at Bruce. His face radiated love and contentment and a certain quality of wonder and excitement. How many years he had walked with his hand in the Saviour's. How long he had searched for just the right church home. As I looked at him the figure of a crippled young man in a wheelchair faded, and I saw a little boy jubilant with his first Vacation Bible School certificate.

Chapter 2

Bruce recovered quickly from surgery. Perhaps the excitement of our new home helped. The rustic log house sat on a hill overlooking Lorane Valley. A boardwalk, hidden beneath a grape arbor, connected an old woodshed to the house. Creeping grapevines twined themselves around every available outcropping and wandered up the west end of the house to curl around Connie's bedroom window. A large barn huddled on a knoll west of the house. Between it and the woodshed wild blackberry vines almost hid an antiquated outhouse. The rise gave way to pastureland that meandered up the hill to an old tumbledown chicken house and a cluster of young fir.

The grove lent its image of mystery to our adventuresome children. Here they could escape from an adult world into fantasy land. The young trees provided hiding places for pirates and Indians. Pioneers solved the problems of a long trek West beneath their sheltering boughs. Sometimes even robbers hunkered in the shadows ready to spring on unsuspecting victims.

An ancient apple orchard clung to the hillside near a spring in a grove of picturesque oak and vine maple. Green apples tempted curious appetites and resulted in several real tummyaches. Above the orchard a forest of stately Douglas fir waved in the breeze until they dropped out of sight over the mountain.

Our new home offered a sketchy view of the small community of Lorane only a mile away. The schools; two stores with gas pumps; the Odd Fellows lodge, which housed the post office; a Grange hall; a few scattered homes; and a nondenominational church made up the village. It was then, and still is, a quaint, beautiful place.

Although religious training was an integral part of our homelife, still we were happy now that the children could go every Sunday to church. While not members of any particular faith, we believed that a family should be well rooted in spiritual knowledge.

The second week after his tonsillectomy Bruce attended church. The gleaming white building, filled nearly to capacity, seemed to beckon to us from the hilltop. The young minister and his wife were friendly. They and the congregation made us feel welcome. Bruce had no qualms about leaving us and going with David to their Sunday School class. After church—where our family, sitting together, occupied a whole pew—Bruce tucked a scribbly-colored picture of Jesus into my hand.

"Here, Mom, keep this. I did it all by myself."

His voice, filled with pride and enthusiasm, made me feel that our new church home had been a good choice. That summer all the children, except the baby, attended Vacation Bible School.

Pleased and completely thrilled, Bruce could hardly wait for its final program. The church invited all the parents and the community to it. The children displayed the crafts they had done. They sang animated choruses and enacted stories from the Bible. The instructors had been especially successful in making the tales from Biblical history meaningful to the several dozen children who participated.

After the final song and benediction, Bruce hurried to us, waving his certificate high overhead.

"Would you carry this for me, Dad? I might tear it, and I don't ever want anything to happen to this. It's a real important certificate!" And it was. It still rests among his keepsakes. The little white church on the hill awakened his spiritual interest.

Due to an uncertain water supply, we could never raise a garden at the old lumber camp shack. Here at Valley View the soil seemed especially eager to grow everything we planted in it. Because they had had a part in raising the garden vegetables, the children ate them with a gusto that was a bit unusual. Bruce particularly enjoyed strawberries. In fact, berries of any sort were his favorite fruits. Wild blackberries, Himalaya berries, and a sweet variety of wild dewberry enticed him to go with anyone of the family that could be persuaded to pick them. All the wild varieties grew profusely on our twelve and a half acres. Some, or all of the family, kept me busy making jams, jellies, and freezing or canning berries for the winter months. Along with the things we preserved from the garden, our storage room bulged at the seams. I almost felt a wave of relief when September came and the children returned to school.

Bruce's health improved so much over the summer months that we decided his problems were over. He had even acquired an enthusiasm for starting to school, an unusual development, for he nearly always began new adventures with skepticism if they meant he would be away from home.

The first day of school dawned bright and clear, with just a hint of fall in the air. Amid all its hustle and bustle Bruce danced from one foot to the other as I tried to comb his hair. Little rivulets of water trickled down his face. I wiped them away with my apron. Never one to do anything halfway, when I had suggested he dampen his hair a bit he had dunked his whole head in the washbasin.

"Please stand still, Bruce!"

"But, Mom, it's almost time for the bus. Can I go by myself with Connie and David?"

"Well, if you'd rather I didn't go——"

"I'd rather, Mom. I'm a big boy now. I even used some of Dad's shaving lotion this morning. Smell it?"

The room reeked with Old Spice. But his courage delighted me, for he had never been this brave when a new situation presented itself. Even his shoulders, which tended to slump, were, with some effort, erect this morning.

"Yes," I agreed, "all little boys need shaving lotion their first day of school." He grinned at me and wrinkled his nose.

"Smells good, huh?"

"Indeed it does. And you may go by yourself if you wish. Just let Connie or David help you find your room."

When the school bus pulled up to our driveway he stood waiting. Sandwiched between Connie and David, he struggled up the steep steps and found a seat by a window. As the bus drove away he waved to where I watched from the front porch. Already that unruly lock of hair strayed from a wet wave and drooped over one eye.

Bruce loved his teacher. An outgoing, pleasant person, she made school an adventure. Although not a genius, Bruce did rather well. Proud of his little art projects and various other school papers, he brought them all home for our approval.

The grading system in the Lorane primary grades consisted of Satisfactory +, Satisfactory, and Needs Improvement. It left no room for teacher or parent comments. Bruce had straight Satisfactory's except in writing and art. An S with a minus after it followed those. When I approached Mrs. Whitney about them, she assured me she found no real problem.

"He's just a little careless, Mrs. Wyman. Some children, especially boys, take longer to learn coordination in writing and art. I think you're worrying needlessly."

Was the nagging worry in the back of my mind becoming so noticeable? If so, it didn't make for a good atmosphere for either Bruce or the other children. Back to Dr. Axley I went with my problem.

"You really are concerned about him, aren't you? Well, you've had a right to be. But I think we're over the hump. Give Bruce a year or two of good nutrition and wholesome living, and I'm sure he'll be fine. You know how readily he recovers from everything." He leaned over and patted me. "Now you just stop worrying and take a little time out to enjoy some of the things you like to do. You know that 'all work and no play [made] Jack a dull boy,' and it isn't going to do anything different for Dorothy, either."

After hugging this dear old man, I left the office feeling like a new person. I never saw him alive again. It had been his life's ambition to establish a hospital for Cottage Grove. His dream had come true, but exhausted and drained, his body rebelled. He died suddenly. All South Lane County mourned his death.

Several months after we moved to Valley View, we purchased the property we had been living on. Now we could really call it home. The children grew attached to its beauty and all it had to offer—especially a little fawn that the former owner had raised after its mother met an untimely death. Never confined, she had the run of the place. In spite of my husband's theory that deer were a nuisance and his refusal to let the children claim her for a pet, she wriggled her way into our lives anyway. After an evening when she had crept up behind Lynn, placing her cold nose on the back of his neck while he milked Daisy—our sometimes gentle Jersey cow—he just had to accept her. Although she had frightened him terribly and nearly caused him to spill the milk, her charm overcame him. She loved all of us, but she seemed to have a special rapport with Lynn. I suppose she knew that beneath that gruff surface a gentle man resided. So Bambi came to stay. She adored the children, particularly if they had crackers to share with her. And she preferred to eat from the same bowl with the cat and her kittens, washing all of them thoroughly after a meal. Only Koko, David's little brown dog, had to keep his distance. He never tempted her, for he sensed the damage her sharp hooves could inflict if she became angry. Bambi must have realized that Bruce did things more slowly and with less assurance than the other children. She would lag behind with him if they were hiking up to the orchard or the forest, rubbing against him now and then licking him gently on the face with her little gray tongue.

A frisky young stallion we continued to pasture for our former landlord delighted in racing with the children. Connie and David were old enough to enjoy him, but Bruce liked him only when he could pet or feed him through a protective fence. Never able to run fast, he preferred to go about his own choice of play and gladly leave Skipper to his. Usually the horse stayed high on the mountain, where the feed was best, coming down only when he thought we might offer something special. One day Bruce and David were playing in the fir grove. Skipper's curiosity got the better of him. He trotted down to investigate. For a moment Bruce petted him, but while David played and fondled the young animal, he decided to go back to the house. Probably the horse thought Bruce wanted to race. Whatever his ideas, Skipper ran toward him. In his haste to escape, Bruce lost his balance and sprawled in the dirt. Skipper galloped over him, planting one sharp hoof on Bruce's rib cage, and continued down the hill. Scrambling to his feet, Bruce darted toward the nearest fence for protection. Again he lost his balance as he crawled through the barbed wire. There he hung, helplessly suspended. I could not hear his screams from inside the log house. Connie, playing near the barn, hurried to tell me of his plight. David ran to Bruce's rescue. By the time I reached him, David had picked him off the fence. Whimpering, Bruce staggered down the fence line while keeping his eyes glued to the horse. Mane flying, Skipper shook his head and kicked his heels in the air. He wanted more of the noisy game. I picked up an old board and threw it at him.

"Get back up that hill. You're nothing but a nuisance!"

Skipper dashed away for a few yards, then turned and whinnied his protest. I wiped away Bruce's tears from his dusty face. Blood oozed from a few scratches on his arms.

"Are you all right? Do you hurt anywhere?"

"My arm hurts awful bad!"

Unbuttoning his shirt, I found no blood, but under his left arm a huge gash lay open, exposing tendons and ligaments. David paled and started to speak. I shook my head.

"He's all right, but he may have to have a few stitches. Run and ask Babe if she can take me to town to a doctor." Babe Suiter was our next-door neighbor.

Bruce began crying in earnest. We returned to the house. In a few minutes Babe arrived, and we were on our way to the doctor in Cottage Grove. Connie and David took the little ones to Suiters' house where a neighbor woman offered to watch all the children in both families.

Not since Dr. Axley had passed away had we needed a doctor. But the new hospital had drawn several physicians to the community. Two of them were Seventh-day Adventists who had established their practice together in a small clinic. Years before, when we had lived in Baker, Oregon, and again in Portland, we had had Adventist doctors. We had found them compassionate and qualified. So I chose to take Bruce to Dr. Stanton G. Oberg. Quiet and reserved, he was not at all inclined to discuss various subjects outside the realm of medicine as Dr. Axley had been. However, he seemed thorough, kind, and considerate. And young—considering the fatherly gray-haired man our beloved Dr. Axley was. Even so, he had a warm smile and a most efficient bedside manner.

He examined Bruce's injuries carefully. Fortunately Bruce had no broken ribs as I had feared. Then Dr. Oberg explained in detail why a cut in that area of the arm did not bleed profusely and of the danger of infection it could entail.

Bruce listened bravely while the doctor told him he would have to take a few stitches in his underarm. The injection of an anesthetic into the muscle made him wince, but he didn't cry. Sometimes he seemed too courageous for a little boy only seven when he faced illness or injury.

After a tetanus shot and a sling arranged to keep the arm immobile, we prepared to leave. Dr. Oberg reached down to Bruce and ruffled his hair. "Be careful of those barbed-wire fences, Bruce. They can be pretty vicious."

Bruce grinned and promised he would, then dashed for the car, eager to tell Babe all about his stitches. As I paid the receptionist and turned to leave I thought of the doctor's camaraderie with my son. The mannerism gave me a welcome feeling.

That evening, after the children were all in bed, I approached my husband.

"Please call Alton and have him come get Skipper. He's really going to hurt someone, he's such a roughneck."

"Right you are!" Lynn walked to the telephone and called the horse's owner immediately. In a few days he came after him. So Skipper rode out of our lives. Although our family, with the exception of Nova, loved horses, we weren't sorry to see that one leave. Now the children could run and play to their hearts' content with nothing more than lovable Bambi to worry about.

Chapter 3

Bruce's second-grade teacher was motherly and completely dedicated to her charges. Connie and David had both been in her room through their first and second grades. Bruce seemed much at ease under her tutoring. His grades remained about the same, with the usual minuses after art and writing.

One January morning, shortly after the children had left for school, the telephone rang. Mrs. Hanns' voice on the line sounded concerned. "Mrs. Wyman, I wonder if you could come down to the school sometime this week? I'd like very much to speak with you about a matter concerning Bruce."

"Is there something wrong, Mrs. Hanns?"

"Well, I'm not really sure. Bruce is such a lovely child, but I feel he has coordination problems. I'd rather not discuss it on the phone. Could you come see me?"

Promising her I would be down that afternoon, I replaced the telephone in its cradle as cold chills crept up my spine. *We've been so certain he looks, feels, and acts better. Mrs. Hanns must surely be imagining things.* But even as I tried to convince myself, I knew it was just wishful thinking. He still fell as often as ever, and each year his shoulders stooped a little more, so I could not make myself believe that his muscles were any less tense than they had been for years.

I timed my arrival at school just before the afternoon recess. Curious children gathered about me, and Bruce hung onto my arm. Mrs. Hanns deftly steered them all out to play. As we sat down on two miniature chairs to talk, I could see the anxiety in her eyes.

"Perhaps I'm making mountains out of molehills, Mrs. Wyman, but I definitely feel that Bruce is not developing normally."

"Can you explain in a little more detail, Mrs. Hanns?"

"Certainly." She described what she felt to be abnormal. Bruce could not make letters or figures accurately, not because he didn't know how, but rather because he could not manipulate his fingers properly. Mrs. Hanns was aware of the tenseness of his muscles and his frequent stumbling and falling. But more than anything she was concerned about his reluctance to try the exercises that children his age delighted in performing.

"It is not that Bruce doesn't understand how to do them. He just has a fear of trying because he realizes that he simply cannot execute the actions with the ease the other children do. Naturally he doesn't want to feel that he is any different, and he certainly doesn't want to be ridiculed. You know how cruel children can be to one another."

"Yes, I do. Would you recommend professional examination?"

"I most certainly do. There is no doubt in my mind at all that Bruce needs special assistance."

Since she was a teacher with excellent qualifications and many years of experience, we could not ignore her advice. After much discussion we decided to take him to our family physician first. Dr. Oberg examined him thoroughly and put him through numerous coordination tests.

"I definitely agree with Bruce's teacher," he said after Bruce had left the room. "His muscular coordination and nerve reflexes are very impaired. But with only this simple examination, I know that it is out of my line. I think you should take him to a specialist, a pediatrician first that I know to be interested and qualified to make a diagnosis. She will know where to send him after that."

The appointment with a pediatrician in Eugene, Oregon, began a long series of trips to specialists. Dr. Tingle's investigation corroborated Dr. Oberg's. She looked at my husband and me with deep concern on her face.

"I see much here that is not as it should be. Bruce's neuromuscular coordination is bad. Please do not be unduly alarmed, for with my knowledge and equipment I cannot be certain. But it is my opinion that perhaps your son has a brain tumor or some obstruction that is impeding the nerve impulses to the muscles. I would like to make an appointment for him with Dr. Robert Dow, who is affiliated with the University of Oregon Medical School in Portland."

Dr. Tingle had said, "Do not be unduly alarmed." She might as well have said, "Do not breathe for the next half hour." Feeling a cold knot twist in my stomach, I looked at Lynn. His expression was blank, and I knew that her words had left him speechless. His son, this dark-skinned little creature he loved so much, could not possibly have anything as wrong with him as a brain tumor. His voice broke the silence.

"Are you certain?"

"No, I'm not certain he has a tumor. I am just certain he has a neuromuscular problem, and I think he should see a neurologist."

No one could deny her honesty or her concern. We asked her to make the appointment.

In February we took Bruce to Portland. The season was rainy and cold. We left home in the wee hours of the morning, making a bed for Bruce in the back seat so he would not be tired when we arrived at the medical school. However, with his usual excitement and curiosity, he didn't sleep a wink. He was convinced the trip would be a real adventure.

Dr. Dow made us feel welcome even in a strange atmosphere. An older man with graying hair and a pleasant smile, he adeptly eased our tensions. He had a whole staff of assistants at his command. We lost count of the various young doctors who examined Bruce and took long sheets of notes on his history and the background of both sides of our family. They asked us to remember every minute detail of anything unusual that had happened to Bruce. His abnormal birth, the high fever the winter we'd been snowbound, the fall from the old fir tree, the experience with the horse Skipper, and a long list of other incidents seemed to hold special significance to all the specialists. They drew large quantities of blood for tests too numerous to remember and X-rayed his body from head to toes.

In probing Bruce's skull with his fingers one young man commented to him, "Well, Bruce, you are part Indian, aren't you?"

My son beamed. He had always been proud of the fact that Lynn's Indian ancestry showed more in him than any of our children. "Yep, but how did you know?"

"From the formation of the head bones. We Indians have a special mark of identification. Feel that slight ridge that runs across the top of your head?"

I saw Lynn reach up to feel his own head. While I had always known that Bruce had the ridge, I had never given it any consideration. My son rubbed his hand across his head.

"Sure thing, I've got one!"

"Of course you have. Know what tribe you're from?"

"Yep, Cherokee. My great-grandfather was raised by the Indians." There was no mistaking the pride in his voice.

"Me, too! Did you know our ancestors were the only tribe that had a written language?" Thereupon began a long conversation between a little boy and a young neurologist about the American Indian. In the process he wrangled all sorts of information out of Bruce about how various things affected him and how he felt.

Late in the afternoon Dr. Dow approached us. "Do you have accommodations in town? We're going to have to run extensive tests on Bruce, and it will take about three days for the results. Tomorrow we'd like to do a spinal-fluid test and run an electroencephalogram."

We had no idea what most of the tests were all about, but we assured him we would be on hand when they needed our son. Previously we had made arrangements to stay with one of my nieces, who had two boys about Bruce's age.

The next morning, after an enjoyable evening with our family, we returned to the medical school. The doctors discouraged us from watching the taking of the spinal fluid. "It's quite painful, and we just think it's better this way." So they whisked Bruce away on a stretcher, and I listened for his screams, a huge lump in my throat. But they never came. A half hour or so later they wheeled him back, Bruce all smiles and talking with the nurses. The doctor pursed his lips and shook his head.

"I can't believe this boy. He's just plain got guts! He never shed a tear or let out a peep. Usually at this age they scream to high heaven."

"A-aw, it didn't hurt much." Bruce had made up his mind to be brave, and he wasn't about to back down yet.

For the electroencephalogram we had to go to another building several blocks away. Here in a neat little room they fitted Bruce with a crown of needles attached to a set of wires that led to a recording machine. For the first time he showed signs of apprehension. He did look weird, like pictures from a science-fiction book of some strange outer-space creature. The attendant realized his fear and explained the whole process to him.

"This won't hurt a bit, Bruce. All these little needles and wires are going to tell us what goes on inside your head. It will all be registered with the needle on this funny-looking roll of paper. In fact, you're going to do something I'll bet none of the rest of your family has ever done. You're going to write a book. And you won't even need a pen!"

Bruce looked at her as if he wasn't quite sure she had all her faculties, but he promised he would do exactly as she asked.

Electroencephalograms were rather new at that time and were performed differently than they are now. The technicians had Bruce do stress exercises and various other procedures that recorded the function of his brain in relation to the nerves and muscles. It took more than two hours. Exhaustion enveloped his body and sweat stood out on his forehead when the nurse finally told him they were through. She showed him the rolls and rolls of squiggly needle marks he had done. Bruce muttered something and seemed anxious to leave.

The sun had come out, and the air felt refreshing as we walked back to the original offices. Bruce was strangely quiet. When his father asked him what troubled him, he replied, "I know I really did write a book—a great big, long one—but for the life of me I don't see how anyone is ever going to read it!"

We spent much of the three days of examination trying to keep Bruce amused while we waited hour after hour in one reception room or another. Finally Dr. Dow came to us and asked if we wouldn't prefer seeing some of the sights Portland had to offer.

"We really won't need you anymore now until all of the lab work is completed. There's no need for you to sit in these boring offices. Is there a telephone number where I can reach you? After all, Portland is a rather lovely place, we think, and we'd like Bruce to think so too."

With genuine relief we gave him my niece's number, and Bruce became excited over the prospect of a trip to the Portland zoo. The weather didn't cooperate well, but we decided not to let the rain interfere with a chance to see the hundreds of interesting animals in Oregon's largest zoo.

Bruce thrilled at the size and antics of the various creatures. His greatest interests were the camels and dromedaries. A congenial zoo attendant explained all the differences between the two and even offered to let him ride a camel. Bruce declined, not from fear, but because the thought of getting on that dripping wet, hairy animal was a bit too much even for a curious boy. The stench of its coat nauseated all of us. Despite the damp fur, I believe Bruce would have attempted a ride, but he couldn't quite stomach the idea of roaming about the rest of the zoo in stinky, wet clothes, for we had no change in the car for him. He wasn't about to give up the excitement of seeing all the other animals for just a little ride on an old camel.

The third day we went back to the medical clinic for the results of the tests and the doctors' conclusions. While Bruce played in a reception room with a little boy about his age who moved about rather well on crutches we talked privately with Dr. Dow.

"I'm sure you people will be happy and relieved to know that we can find no positive results to any of the numerous tests we've run on Bruce to see if he has a brain tumor. There is one more procedure we could initiate, but I do not advise it at this time. That is an angiogram. It is very risky and extremely painful. There simply is not, in my opinion, any reason to subject Bruce to this. If he were my son, I would allow it only as a last resort and then only if all the other examinations proved beyond reasonable doubt that he had a tumor."

A wave of relief washed over me. Somehow the words *brain tumor* had frightened me beyond description. A relaxed sigh escaped from Lynn. Although he had never admitted to being afraid of the idea, I knew now that it had bothered him. Dr. Dow must have recognized our reaction. He smiled.

"Now I don't want you to be overly encouraged," and a frown furrowed his brow. "Bruce definitely has something wrong neurologically. But we don't think it is a brain tumor."

"Have you found something else?" I was almost afraid to ask, for perhaps there were many things worse than tumors.

"That is the sixty-four-dollar question, Mrs. Wyman. We haven't been able to pinpoint any reason for Bruce's problem. There is a problem, please don't misunderstand me. His muscles do not receive the proper nerve impulses, but in all honesty, I must tell you that we don't know why. Neuromuscular ailments are extremely complex, and to be perfectly frank, medical science is quite inadequate at this point. But we are trying hard to learn—there's just an awful lot we don't know."

I found myself liking him for many reasons, but especially for his honesty.

My husband, always practical, looked serious. "Are you saying all these examinations have been for nothing?"

"Not at all, for we have come up with some interesting conclusions. But surely you would not want me to tell you I know exactly what Bruce's problem is when in all honesty I do not."

Lynn looked chagrined. "No, of course not. I'm sorry."

"Don't be sorry for your feelings for one minute, Mr. Wyman. You have every right to be skeptical. Your son has just been subjected to a lot of misery, and this sort of thing, I'm sure you already know, is not bought with peanuts."

Immediately Lynn felt at ease. "Well, what can you tell us then, Doctor?"

"I could go into a lot of medical phraseology, which I'm sure wouldn't mean much to you at this point, but I'm not going to. To break it down in plain English, we believe that Bruce has suffered brain damage for some reason, probably the excessively high fever he experienced when he had tonsillitis. Or it could have been the fall from the tree. Or it may have been simply a quirk of nature. But whatever the cause, we feel encouraged that the consequences will lessen as he learns to live with the situation. We believe that whatever the damage is, it will not get any worse."

His words, spoken with honest conviction, thrilled us. We must have looked at him as if he had performed some sort of miracle.

"Don't for one minute think your problems are over. Bruce will never be just exactly like his brother and sisters or his friends. You'll run into all sorts of emotional and physical enigmas, especially behavioral puzzles. But don't let them throw you. And by all means, keep his life normal among his family and his peers. Never let him get away with things you would not allow your other children to do, since his responsibilities are just as great as anyone else's. Make him feel needed and let him know often that his place in the home is just as important as is any other member's in the family group. I cannot emphasize this too much! Above all, love him."

The organ reverberated through the church as the organist broke into the opening chords of "Shall We Gather at the River?" The congregation rose as one. Their voices pealed forth in praise while the words "Where bright angel feet have trod" rang through the room. Tony motioned for my husband to wheel Bruce forward as other attendants opened the baptistry. Bruce's face was radiant. Tony slipped off my son's shoes, and he and another assistant lifted him from the wheelchair and carried him to the edge of the pool, where they eased his crippled body down into the heated water. Without willing them to do so, Bruce's muscles automatically tightened as they always had when confronted with water. Forewarned, Tony spoke a comforting phrase to him, and Bruce relaxed in his arms. As they lowered him into the water my eyes blurred, and I saw again a frightened little boy trying so hard to act brave when his swimming instructor lifted him into a blue pool where dozens of children romped in glee.

Chapter 4

How true Dr. Dow's words proved to be! Little more than a week had gone by since we returned from Portland when the first behavior riddle presented itself. Bruce threw a tantrum—a genuine, uninhibited, screaming, kicking tantrum. I can't recall the circumstances that triggered it, but I can well remember his reaction. One of the children had done some small thing that angered him. Instead of the usual slaps or yells, Bruce clenched his fists at his sides. His whole body shook. As he held his breath, his face turned a purple-red, and he glared at the other child. Connie stared in disbelief, her mouth hanging open.

I stopped folding bath towels on the dining table. "Bruce, stop that this instant!"

As if my voice had released a brake, Bruce screamed at the top of his voice and flung himself on the floor, kicking his feet as fast and hard as he could against the floor or whatever else happened to get in his way. For a moment I feared some sort of convulsion, because Bruce had never behaved that way before. And then I saw that in spite of all the noise and contortions, he stole glances at me out of the corner of squinted eyes. I remembered Dr. Dow's warning—*you'll run into all sorts of emotional and behavioral puzzles.* Yet I couldn't imagine what Bruce thought he might gain by his actions. But I also remembered—*never let him get away with things you would not allow your other children to do.* Still I felt apprehensive about the whole situation. Grasping him by one flailing arm, I asked, "Brucie, what is the matter? Don't be like this."

It only made him scream louder and kick harder. Anger flared within me. I picked him up, laid him over the arm of the couch, and applied the palm of my hand to the seat of his pants with several good, hard whacks. Then I carried him across the room and sat him firmly on a straight-backed chair.

"Now, young man, you sit there until you can behave yourself, and I don't want to hear one word out of you until then. When you think you can be good, we'll talk about what happened."

The tantrum ceased. Bruce, who usually bellowed loudly if spanked, only whimpered. In a few minutes he sat, quiet and pouty. Although he was always one to look another direct in the eye, when I spoke to him he kept his eyes lowered.

"Bruce," I repeated, "I asked you a question. Why did you act like that?"

Slowly he raised his head, big tears spilling down his cheeks. "I don't know. It just seemed like a good idea."

"Well, believe me, Son, it wasn't."

I had to busy myself with the clothes-folding to repress a chuckle. How well I remembered another time when he was about four and had kept me up all night with a make-believe earache because he couldn't sleep. When I asked him why he had done it, he had given me the same answer: "I don't know. It just seemed like a good idea."

We discussed the virtues of controlling tempers and living by the Golden Rule and how it makes our heavenly Father sad when we act naughty. When I felt I had gotten the point across, I told him to run and play. That whimsical smile played at the corners of his mouth. With a quick hug and a promise he'd never do it again, he ran outside. I can't say that it didn't happen again. Sometimes little boys' promises get lost in the shuffle. It occurred quite frequently for the next two or three years, although he well knew what the consequences would be each time. Somehow all the sessions in doctors' offices made him realize—in a subconscious way—that he encountered difficulties the other children didn't. He began to think we should pamper him. When we didn't, the tantrums came. Perhaps they released frustrations with which he couldn't otherwise cope.

Before school closed in May, the parents in the community made arrangements to use the school bus to transport children to swimming lessons three times weekly at Drain, Oregon. Connie and David had already had a year or two of instruction. Now the time had arrived for Bruce to learn to swim. But, reluctant and uneasy, he begged not to go. We insisted.

One day, as I watched from the sidelines, a chubby boy I didn't know approached me. "Are you Bruce's mamma?"

"Yes."

"How come he gets to dog-paddle and the rest of us don't?"

I informed the little boy I hadn't the vaguest idea, but that I would find out. When I confronted the swimming instructor he told me it was not routine, but because Bruce had difficulty kicking his legs properly, he felt that dog-paddling would at least keep him from drowning if the situation ever arose. While I could understand his viewpoint, I still wanted my son to learn to swim properly.

"I realize that, Mrs. Wyman," he said. "True, we are here to teach these children to swim, but we are also here to help them keep from drowning. In Bruce's case I feel this is of prime importance. We are teaching him all the other procedures, but it's going to take time with him. He has an unusual fear of water but more determination than most to conquer it. Perhaps my method is a little out of the ordinary, but I think it is important to Bruce."

I couldn't argue the point with him. Besides, who was I—who couldn't swim a stroke—to question a qualified instructor? The instructor swam over to Bruce, who sat on the edge of the pool. He held out his arms. My son tried to ease himself into the water, but his muscles tensed, and he shivered. The teacher gathered him into his arms and helped him paddle along the poolside. As they passed in front of me I heard him say, "Remember, Bruce, the water is your enemy only when you are afraid of it. When you are relaxed and ready to have fun, it's your friend." Bruce grinned, rolled over on his stomach, and bravely tried to swim several strokes. When he had reached the limit of his endurance, the instructor lifted him out of the water and swung him high.

"Good boy, you're getting better all the time." He eased him down on a paddleboard. "Now let me see you practice those leg kicks." As Bruce paddled away he turned and, with a wink of his eye, gave me an OK gesture with his thumb and forefinger.

As long as we lived in Lorane, Bruce continued taking swimming instruction every summer.

Life at Valley View became rather routine. Lynn continued to work in Cottage Grove, and things went along much the same each season. Nine months of school alternated with summer times full of Vacation Bible School sessions, swimming lessons, gardening, and all sorts of fun times. We experienced sad events, funny situations, and sometimes frightening ones. But they all comprised part of the growing process of a large family. Only the tragic death in a logging accident of our beloved Ken, Nita's husband, shattered the children's lives. All of us mourned his passing, but Bruce sobbed uncontrollably. It took a long while to coax him into a state of acceptance. He loved Ken and couldn't imagine life without him. But five weeks later, when Nita gave birth to her first son—little Ken—all of the children, including Bruce, transferred their love for Ken to the squirming, tiny image of their adored cousin.

Appointments with the dentist or doctor, bouts with flu and colds, Christmases with their accompanying school programs, Valentine parties, church activities, and spring vacations kept us a busy, occupied family.

Just before Christmas, 1953, we received an early present. Tiny, black-haired Danna Layne came to live with us. All of the children considered her a precious gift. But try as hard as they could not to show it, Bruce and David couldn't hide their disappointment. They had wanted a baby brother so badly. Talking to me on the phone, while I rested in the hospital, Bruce sounded tearful.

"What's the matter, Bruce?"

"But, Mom, I wanted her to be a boy!"

Reasons a little girl should make him happy raced through my mind.

"Bruce, I'm sure a boy couldn't possibly have looked as much like you as this little girl does. She's got your dark eyes and a whole mop of black hair just like you had when you were born." Silence hung on the line. "Did you hear me, Bruce?"

"Are you kiddin', Mom?"

"Not a bit. She is just a tiny Bruce, only she's a girl."

"Hey, you guys, listen," he called to anyone close enough to hear. "Mom says the baby looks just like me. Did you hear that, Grandma? The baby looks just like me!"

For once I had managed to say the right thing. About two weeks after I came home with the baby, I gave her to David to hold while I warmed a bottle. Never one to let anyone know about his sentimentality, I heard him whisper to the little bundle in his arms, "We wouldn't trade you for a dozen boys, would we?"

When Lynn was a child, he had lived in the eastern Oregon cattle and lumber town of Lakeview. He never ceased to love its seclusion and dry high-desert climate. Afflicted with asthma and hay fever from the lush vegetation of Lane County, he treasured the chance to go deer hunting each fall in eastern Oregon. He would come home with clear eyes and minus his usual sinus infection.

One such fall he returned with excitement in his eyes. "What would you say if I suggested that we move to Lakeview?"

He waited for me to explode. Actually his words came as no surprise. I knew how he liked the wide, open spaces, and I rather envied his hunting trips. Sometimes I, too, felt lonely for open country, having been raised in the sagebrush area of southern Idaho.

"Sounds great," I said. "What do you propose we do for a living?"

Unable to hide his enthusiasm, he told me of a big ranch whose owner wanted to lease his grain acreage and machinery to someone. A victim of polio, the rancher had decided to try life in town as a car salesman while still operating his cattle business. I had qualms about being able to maintain our household without a monthly income, but the climate might prove a drawing card not only for Lynn and his asthmatic condition but for Nova Lynne and her constant battle with colds and infected tonsils. I was willing to sacrifice a good deal for that.

The boys were thrilled. They had accompanied their father on the hunting excursions once or twice, and the desert country of Oregon fascinated them, too. It didn't matter much to Nova and Merrie, but Connie was crushed. She felt certain she could never make new friends nor leave her old ones. But adventure won, and we moved the first of November, 1954, to Drews Valley and Hay Creek Ranch.

Regarding Bruce, it seemed like a risky thing to do. It meant changing doctors. However, Dr. Oberg didn't consider it hazardous, since the specialists all agreed that his condition would not worsen. "Any qualified physician can handle his case now, and I will be glad to transfer his records at any time."

That settled it. Besides, we really couldn't see that his state of health showed either much improvement or deterioration since the trip to Portland in 1952. Although his muscles didn't seem any less tense and his shoulders continued to slump, he had learned to hop on one foot, something he could never accomplish before.

Since we were inclined to grasp at straws concerning his improvement, it excited all of us.

If our house at Valley View had seemed immense, the one at Hay Creek Ranch was gargantuan. A white three-story square structure, built in the early 1900s for a sort of hotel and stage stop, it had seven bedrooms on the second floor. Never used for its original purpose, the third floor remained just an outsized attic. The ground floor had a large living room and two bedrooms. Merrie Jo and baby Danna shared one, and Lynn and I occupied the larger one. Upstairs the other children could each have his own room. But Connie and Nova chose a room together. A long hallway ran downstairs. On the second floor a wide staircase with an ornate carved railing provided an ideal setting for romantic young girls to make dramatic entries to pretend weddings or theater productions. In it also once hung an effigy to frighten the girls, the brainchild of Bruce and David and a boyfriend. The kitchen, spacious and inviting, produced heat for chilled bodies and for all our cooking from an old-fashioned black wood range that stood stalwart and unyielding in one corner. A long homemade dining table, which could easily seat twenty people, rambled along one wall. Lengthy hand-carpentered benches on both sides of the table made seating room. And wonder of wonders, off the kitchen was an honest-to-goodness, genuine, pink-and-black bathroom, complete with gleaming white tub and separate shower stall. And it actually worked. It seemed too good to be true. When Connie saw it, she lost all despair about our move.

The boys leaped at the chance to learn farming with their father, and so did Nova Lynne. We had horses to ride, cattle to feed, cows to milk, fields to plow and seed, pigs to care for, and bummer lambs to nurse through babyhood. Bruce especially enjoyed riding a stubborn black Shetland-Welch crossbred pony named Champ. After dumping Bruce unceremoniously several times into the little creek that gurgled through the barnyard and wandered past the house, Champ and Bruce finally reached an understanding and became fast friends.

However, we also had sacrifices to make and hardships to overcome in our new venture. We were used to Lane County, where the temperature seldom got much below freezing. Here the first winter the thermometer plunged to thirty-three degrees below zero, with a high wind off Drews Reservoir that increased the chill factor. Snow piled deep. It took a bit of getting used to for all of us. But it gave the children a chance to learn to ice-skate and ski, though Bruce never mastered either, and they all learned survival in an unpredictable climate.

A daily bus ride of twenty miles to and from school, with a half-mile hike to the bus stop, presented a real battle for Bruce. Slow and clumsy in the deep snow, he often kept a patient bus driver waiting. Bruce never complained, except for the cold. That was difficult for him to adjust to, for his slower movements invited cold hands and feet. But he never used it as an excuse not to go to school.

The distance to town meant we had to give up a lot of social events, and church was an infrequent pleasure. We compensated by doing things together as a family. Lynn and I concentrated on acquainting the children with Bible stories and spiritual lessons that they could apply to their everyday living. But we took them to town to various activities as often as our finances permitted.

David and Bruce began hunting and fishing together.

Drews Valley, a sportsman's Utopia, abounded with waterfowl and fishing streams. Bruce would sit for hours on the bank of a stream to fish or on a rocky butte waiting for a flock of geese. He brought home his share of the bag limit too.

My misgivings about the financial status of our move proved legitimate—we nearly lost our proverbial shirts. But because of our poverty, the family drew closer together. We learned lessons of love and skill that would otherwise have been unlikely. Through our own creativity we made what we could not afford to buy. And what we couldn't make, we did without. Minus social luxuries and television, the children became avid readers. They soon learned that the covers of a book hid untold worlds of adventure and imagination. We often shared books and read aloud to the entire family.

Connie's worries about making new friends proved groundless. All the children acquired numerous ones, and the house sheltered one or another of them nearly every weekend. Despite our isolation, we had droves of company and never suffered from loneliness.

Bruce did rather well in school through the fifth and sixth grades, thanks to two especially understanding teachers. But the seventh grade in junior high presented quite another situation. There he had to climb stairs to his various classes. They were difficult for him to negotiate. Most of his teachers gave him every encouragement. But he had one science teacher who undid all the progress the others made possible. Arrogant and impatient, he refused to correct Bruce's papers. When confronted with the fact, he insisted that my son was retarded, sloppy, uncooperative, and not worth a teacher's time or effort. Up until then none of Bruce's teachers had ever given us any reason to believe he reacted in that manner to his schoolwork. I demanded to see recent IQ and aptitude tests, to which parents, at that time, were not allowed access. The man relented and let me see them. Both to his surprise and mine—for he hadn't bothered to consult them—Bruce's IQ showed far above average. His aptitudes did leave something to be desired, because he could not cope with normal circumstances expected of others his age. The teacher did back down and agree to correct Bruce's work and do what he could to help him, but he did so reluctantly. His actions toward Bruce discouraged the boy more than anything anyone had ever done to him up to that time. He has never fully recovered from the humiliation. That teacher's attitude certainly made us aware that a good teacher is worth many times over his or her salary, and a poor one isn't worth a dime of it.

In the fall of 1957 our lease expired on the ranch. Since its owner hadn't been any more successful as a car salesman than we had at ranching, he and his family wanted to come home. Renewing our lease was out of the question.

We rented a cozy home in the little ranching and farming community of West Side and moved into it on a stormy November day. Although we felt sad about leaving the ranch we loved so much, we were consoled by the fact that the Tracys, who owned it, were among our best friends. And we still owned Valley View. But the absence of hay fever, sinus infections, rampant colds, and tonsillitis was something we weren't willing to give up. As a result we all elected to remain in eastern Oregon. Besides, Connie and David were close to high school graduation, and Connie, thoroughly infatuated with a local boy, adamantly refused to leave Lake County.

In a matter of a few days Lynn went to work for Weyerhaeuser Company as a heavy-duty mechanic. Although the job required his staying in a woods camp through the week, we all felt secure again with his steady income. His absence made the weekends when he came home seem like holidays or special occasions.

Connie and David continued at Lakeview High School, but Bruce, Nova, and Merrie Jo attended Union, a small country elementary school near our home. Bruce bubbled with excitement. Certain that the new school would be easier to cope with, he felt it an answer to his prayers. His enthusiasm was short-lived. His eighth-grade teacher must have been cast from the same mold as his seventh-grade science instructor. Bigoted, contentious, cruel, and uncompromising, he couldn't even get along with his own daughter, who shared the same class. He had little patience with my son.

Bruce's eighth-grade graduation, which should have been a triumph, turned out to be a tragic occasion. Since the school had no auditorium, it held the closing exercises in the local Grange hall. A small decorated rostrum seated part of the school board, the teacher, and the speaker of the evening. The students sat in the first row of the audience and marched up a rickety flight of steps to receive their diplomas. After a congratulatory handshake they went down equally unstable stairs back to their seats. Some of the boys asked if one of them or an attendant could help Bruce when his turn came. The teacher refused. *Bruce would not receive any special favors and would do exactly as the other boys did.* Unaware of the situation, neither my husband nor I interceded. When Bruce went up to accept his diploma, we held our breath and prayed, not wanting to embarrass him by showing our concern. I could sense the boys in his class doing the same thing. As Bruce started down the first step he lost his balance and fell full length on the bare, varnished floor below. The chairman of the school board rushed to his aid. But before he could reach him, one of the graduating boys, without bothering to ask permission from anyone, ran forward and helped him to his feet. Face flushed and embarrassment covering him like a cloak, Bruce stumbled to his seat. A compassionate moan escaped the audience. Lynn and I sat crushed with the humiliation we knew enshrouded our son. His teacher never offered to assist him but sat on the rostrum, his face engulfed in a smirking grin. The entire evening lost some of its glamour, not only for Bruce and his family, but for his friends and the parents gathered there for the occasion.

But Bruce's antagonistic teacher was only one thorn in an otherwise outstanding community. Bruce made a host of loving and kind friends at West Side. Mike, Doug, Jay, and Linny were only a few of those who watched over him unceasingly and have continued to keep in touch with him. Norma, the school cook and custodian, took him under her wing and made sure he never missed the important things. He encountered the unlimited interest and love of a dedicated Scout master. Through Ralph Patrick's perseverance, Bruce attended Boy Scout camp at Crescent Lake, where he struggled until he had earned his Scout badge in swimming. A Conservative Baptist youth camp offered a chance for spiritual development and interesting friendships. The minister—a big, blustery overgrown cowboy—and his thoughtful wife promoted love and warmth in Christian gatherings and always took Bruce with them to various church excursions. It was here he really began to realize that God occupied an important part in his life. He and the minister and his family became extremely close.

With church attendance once again possible on a frequent basis for Bruce, he reached a new awareness of Christ in his life. He began to realize that every individual must make his own commitment to spiritual responsibility. No longer could he slide by on what his mother and father taught or what their personal beliefs were. Instead, he must make up his own mind. Accepting Christ into his life as his personal Saviour presented no problem for Bruce. Perhaps his lack of ability to participate in all the activities common to his age group strengthened his desire to put his trust in God. Or perhaps it was just a manifestation of his own unique personality. Whatever compelled him, he gave his heart to the Lord during his early teenage years through the leadership of his friend Al, the cowboy preacher.

But Bruce had always possessed a curious mind. He could never be satisfied with a "this is just the way it is" kind of an answer. Rather he had to know the why, what, when, and where about everything. Religion was no exception. Although he enjoyed attending the little West Side Conservative Baptist church, he would not officially become a member of its congregation.

"I won't join any church until I am satisfied it is the one for me," he insisted. He kept that promise to himself.

In October, 1958, just after he entered high school, Bruce returned to Portland and Dr. Dow. For a number of years he had been under the care of Dr. Paul Kliewer in Lakeview. Kliewer was dissatisfied with Bruce's progress. It had become quite evident that the handicap had not lessened as he learned to live with it, but rather he became steadily more incapacitated as the years went by. Whatever afflicted Bruce relaxed its impact on his body during his boyhood, but as he grew into a teenager the disease gripped his nerves and muscles with more power and speed than ever before during his life.

"This handicap is beyond my medical comprehension," Dr. Kliewer said to me one late August day after he had given Bruce his required high school entry physical examination. "You know, and so do I, that Bruce's general health is exceptionally good, but this neuromuscular ailment is fast making a cripple of him. I'd like him to go through the neurological clinic again. New things are being discovered every day, and Bruce should have the advantage of anything, no matter how small, that could possibly help him."

Lynn and I agreed, but it took two months to get an appointment.

The clinic hadn't changed much. Dr. Dow seemed a little older, perhaps a little grayer, but he was still the straightforward person we'd learned to know back in 1952. However, a new set of doctors had replaced the ranks of his staff as the former ones had gone their separate ways.

Bruce underwent all the same tests and examinations, plus a few new ones given him the first time through the clinic. Some of the techniques had changed considerably. It again took three days to complete them. While Bruce discussed his case with a young neurosurgeon, Dr. Dow spoke with us in his private office.

"I wish I could give you people some real encouragement, but I can't. We haven't yet been able to pinpoint a cause for Bruce's condition. We've been forced to change our opinions about a lot of things. I felt so certain when he was small that the brain-cell deterioration would not progress. But it has, and at rather a rapid pace." He arose from his desk and for a few moments paced the floor, then stared quietly out the window at distant Mt. Hood. I sensed a sadness in his attitude. After a long silence, he returned to his desk.

"It's frustrating to have a patient who so desperately needs your help, and you can't give him any." I knew the feeling well and could sympathize with his sense of futility.

"Bruce's motor nerve cells are deteriorating, as nearly as we can determine, much in the same manner as occurs in old age. But we haven't the vaguest idea why. There is one bright spot. He has a phenomenal mind. We're very fortunate that it is neuromuscular rather than mental. It could have gone either way. It is my opinion that he will eventually be totally handicapped. I can't say how long it will take."

Suddenly it seemed as if the office walls would collapse and crush me. *No, no, no, it isn't true. They just haven't found the cause. This can't happen to my Bruce!* But I knew in my heart that the doctor's words were nothing more than echoes of the fears I had long pushed into the dark recesses of my mind and refused to accept. Lynn sat silent, impassive. Would he believe the finality of the doctor's opinion? He had never conceded to his son's being a cripple, nor would he allow anyone else to. At last he broke the silence, and his words surprised me.

"If there is no hope, where do we go from here?"

"That's a good question, Mr. Wyman, but I have an answer. Medical science is always searching. We are always, it seems, just on the brink of spectacular discoveries. I'm going to believe, and I hope you will, too, that we'll make one soon that will help Bruce. In the meantime I'd like you to take him now to an orthopedic specialist near here. Bruce's knees and feet are quite misshapen, and they contribute, I feel, to his imbalance. I understand this man has been quite successful. I'd like him to see Bruce."

We made the appointment and went immediately to the orthopedic clinic. People of all sizes, ages, and descriptions, each a victim of some crippling ailment, crowded its reception room. Nurses swished in and out of the room, demanding that this one go here and another there. No one seemed concerned about the obvious suffering of the patients. *My imagination must be working overtime. I've just been in too many reception rooms, too many offices, seen too many doctors.*

Finally, after a long wait, a nurse ushered us into the doctor's private office. I have long since forgotten his name. Bruce undressed and climbed onto an examination table, and we waited longer for the doctor. Bruce was tired, for it was well into the afternoon. His shoulders slumped even more than usual. At last the physician entered. Small, with hawkish features, he little more than nodded a greeting to us. He walked over to Bruce, doubled his fist, and gave him a firm poke between the shoulder blades.

"Sit up there, boy! What do you think you are, a hunchback?"

It takes one's imagination to believe such an inhuman creature could ever have reached the status of a specialist in any field. In all the years of sessions and consultations with medical people, we had never encountered anyone that could compare with his rudeness. My anger boiled within me. Unable to speak, I walked out of the room. In a darkened hall I broke into tears. I couldn't have treated a dog the way he did my son.

Later Lynn said that when I left the room the doctor followed me with his eyes. He picked up Bruce's file. "Perhaps I'd better look at this boy's records."

Infuriated, Lynn glared at the man. *"Yes, I think you'd better!"*

I never returned to the office. Some time later a nurse escorted us into a tiny stall. Unbelievable as it may seem, that's exactly what it was. Lining one wall of a long, narrow room were stalls, each equipped with a chair and an examination table. In one next to us an elderly couple waited. The man, obviously in much pain, groaned. As a nurse walked by she called him by name and said, "Oh, stop complaining! You're not half as bad off as you think you are."

Lynn looked shocked, and Bruce cringed. It seemed everyone in this place was bent on hurting, not healing. I felt as if we were cattle waiting for slaughter. How had we ever gotten into such a nightmarish situation? Only the fact that the clinic was new and rather unestablished could explain Dr. Dow's sending us there.

After what seemed to us an inadequate examination, Bruce dressed and waited in the same room while the orthopedist talked with us.

"His knees are very impaired. They will never be any better. I recommend that the ligaments be severed. This will straighten his legs, and there will no longer be the pulling of tense muscles." Bruce paled, and his eyes dilated. My husband frowned, his face a mask of disbelief. The specialist continued. "I can make the arrangements today, if you'd like."

I found my voice. "Just a minute, Doctor. If we allow this to be done, Bruce won't be able to walk anymore, will he?"

"Of course not, but it will eliminate the crooked knees. He might as well be in a wheelchair anyway."

Lynn picked up his jacket and helped Bruce off the table. "I don't think we're interested in your proposition." He turned to me. "Come on, let's get out of here."

The doctor looked disappointed. "Well, it's your decision, but I think you're making a mistake."

"I believe, Doctor," I said, "that that is a matter of opinion."

Relief flooded Bruce's features. We stopped at the desk only long enough to pay our bill. As we stepped out into the fall sunshine each of us drew a deep breath of fresh air. I felt as if we had just escaped an execution.

"Dad, did you hear what that doctor said? He wanted to cut the ligaments in my legs!"

"Yes, I heard what he said, and I don't want to discuss it. You just forget all about what he said or did. That man is not a doctor; he's a butcher!"

Bruce recognized his father's anger and dropped the subject. But I saw that capricious grin catch at the corners of his mouth, and his neck muscles bulged as he forced his shoulders to straighten as far as he could.

The rude, unsympathetic doctor had left us cold, bitter, and discouraged. But we returned to Lakeview determined that no one, not even a specialist, would rob our son of even the limited use of his legs he had.

Chapter 5

Bruce returned to school, and life again settled into routine. It became increasingly difficult for him to walk the short distance to catch the bus. Connie, a senior in high school now, always walked beside him, a steadying hand on his arm. In spite of her help, he often fell, sometimes pulling her down with him. The two of them would sit for a moment on the grass or in the snow, laughing together, making a joke out of their predicament, then she'd help him to his feet. With her arm around his waist, they'd make it to the bus, while one of the other children carried their books, lunches, or whatever.

David seemed to feel a sort of embarrassment at Bruce's clumsiness, but he never refused to help him. A junior now, he was quite grown and often elsewhere, involved in sports or various jobs. Connie, as she always had, remained Bruce's champion.

When his records came from the medical clinic, Dr. Kliewer asked us to come into his office for the report. We already knew the general opinions; only the details remained. Dr. Kliewer skipped lightly over the orthopedic report, apparently not agreeing with it any more than we had. We didn't burden him with the gruesome particulars.

"I'd hoped for more than this," he said as he doodled on his desk pad. A tall, angular, athletic type, the doctor showed real compassion for Bruce that was obvious. He, too, had a family. "But, at least, we know now that there is nothing more we can do. You will just have to learn to live with it."

"Doctor," I said, my agitation at him quite apparent, "these dozens of specialists haven't yet found what Bruce has, and you say we are to give up. You're a devout Christian. You well know the power of God. If this were one of your children, would you say the same?"

He bowed his head, and silence hung like a heavy curtain in the room. After a moment he looked at me, eyes misty. Suddenly I felt ashamed that I had forced him to reveal his innermost feelings. But I couldn't take my words back.

Dr. Kliewer cleared his throat. "No, Dorothy, when you put it like that, I guess I wouldn't. We'll continue to search for whatever we can find to help Bruce. Who knows? Maybe some researcher will stumble on something." And he remained true to his word.

The demands of high school, with long flights of stairs to climb and more advanced study courses, proved almost too exhausting for Bruce. His grades fell sharply. The work was not beyond his comprehension—he just didn't have the energy to keep up with his classmates. Nighttime found him overfatigued. He would tumble into bed and sleep almost as if drugged. When morning came, he dragged out of bed, too weary to really care whether he went to school or not.

In spite of his tiredness, he insisted on raising pigs for a 4-H project. Later he would undoubtedly have chosen a different animal, but he had not yet learned the health hazards of pork. David and Nova pitched in to help him. He couldn't display them at the fair, but he did sell them for a reasonable profit.

Moving to West Side didn't stop Bruce from hunting and fishing with David. They went as often as they had time. One day while rabbit hunting, they walked over a rather rough, rocky terrain. David, a sure marksman, slipped along ahead of Bruce, ready for the first shot at some unsuspecting bunny. Suddenly he felt the wind and heard the buzz of something much like the sound of a bee. Fractions of a second later the report of a .22-caliber rifle exploded in his ears. Well trained, David dropped flat to the ground. Silence clung to the afternoon air, broken only by the sough of the wind in the junipers. An anguished cry tore at David's heart. Scrambling to his feet, he ran to Bruce's side. His brother lay in a heap, his gun nearly hidden beneath him.

'Bruce, are you OK?'' No sound escaped his brother's lips and he lay there, his face a ghastly palor. "Bruce, answer me! Are you hit?"

Weak and pale, Bruce struggled to a sitting position. David knelt beside him. A whisper he could scarcely hear broke into a sob. "N-no, I'm all r-right. I—thought—I'd—shot—you!"

David sat on a rock, a protective arm around Bruce's shoulders. "Naw, I'm OK. Pretty close though, huh?"

Hardly able to negotiate the rocky ground, Bruce had stumbled and fallen forward on his gun. Although on safety, either the impact of the fall or a twig of sagebrush displaced it and triggered the rifle. Bruce picked up his gun and handed it butt first to David. "Here, I don't want it anymore. I guess this ends our hunting."

"Oh, no it doesn't! We came out here to hunt rabbits,

and we're going to hunt rabbits! I'll just walk along beside or behind you. Now keep that gun barrel well out in front of you. Come on, let's go."

Where David had picked up his psychology is a mystery. But it eased a traumatic experience for Bruce. When they reached home, a rabbit or two in their pack, David never mentioned the incident. I thought Bruce strangely preoccupied, but dismissed it as fatigue. Cleaning his gun, he carefully placed it on its rack. Several days later he told us of the episode. He seldom went hunting again, except to sit quietly on a stationary stand. From that time on he concentrated on fishing.

Connie graduated in the spring of 1959. During the winter her longtime boyfriend had placed a diamond on her left hand. She and Clyde were married on a sultry July day, Bruce's good friend, the cowboy preacher, officiating. Bruce, I'm sure, wished Connie wouldn't leave home, but he cherished his new brother-in-law. And after all, they were only going as far away as Lakeview.

Clyde belonged to the Assembly of God, and Connie transferred her religious interests there. They came to visit often, frequently taking Bruce to church with them. He became familiar with another approach to religion. Although he enjoyed going, he didn't display any real enthusiasm for the doctrine.

Some time later one of the Lakeview churches held a revival campaign. It was not of their faith, but Connie and Clyde decided to attend. Bruce and I accompanied them. During an altar call, one of the evangelists asked Bruce if he'd like them to pray for him. Never opposed to prayer, Bruce agreed. He wanted so much to be like other boys his age, and he believed in all sincerity that nothing was impossible with God. If divine healing was possible for him, then he wanted it. While I did not feel comfortable with the situation, I didn't want to be guilty of standing in his way.

Although the effort put forth by the evangelist and many others was sincere and compassionate, Bruce did not receive a healing. Perhaps his faith or mine was not strong enough, or that avenue of help did not meet with God's plans for him. Whatever the reason, Bruce didn't allow himself to dwell long on his shattered hopes.

All summer he continued to be exhausted, sleeping until late morning. In the afternoons he would march back and forth across the lawn, trying his best to keep his legs mobile. His lumbering gait tired him. Often he stumbled, catching himself on the yard fence. He would ease himself down in the shade and lie there panting until he felt rested.

Fifteen now, Bruce often longed to have girl friends like his pals had, but he seemed to realize his dreams had little chance of fulfillment. He experienced the same emotional drives as any other young boy but found it necessary to channel them into other areas. He attempted to satisfy the desire for boy-girl relationships by corresponding with a young girl he had played with as a small boy at Valley View. Joan Suiter became his fast friend and confidante. He awaited each of her letters eagerly and kept pictures of her displayed about his room. All of the girls in the Baptist youth group were friends, too, but he never dated them.

September came, and we had to make a decision about school for Bruce. His imbalance had grown much worse. We couldn't trust his safety in the high school building, with its flights of stairs. Already he'd fallen down them a number of times. What saved him from broken limbs was beyond anyone's comprehension. He begged not to go to school, not only because he couldn't manage the steps but because he had reached a stage of development where his handicap left him embarrassed. Dr. Kliewer thought the psychological impact of school for him was too great, to say nothing of the danger to his life. We agreed, although we dreaded the effect the lack of contact with his peers would have on him. Bruce didn't seem happy with the decision to leave school, but he accepted it as just another discomforting consequence of his ailment.

Knowledge, however, one does not necessarily have to gain within the four walls of a school building. After a state-sponsored rehabilitation program turned him down, we considered high school correspondence courses. Neither the county school superintendent nor the doctor agreed with that route. They believed we should channel his energies into hobbies and scientific fields, since his primary interests lay there.

In October the owner sold the house in which we lived. With rentals scarce, we feared we'd have to move to town. None of the family wanted to live in a city. Lakeview, with a population of about three thousand, constituted a city as far as the children were concerned. Merrie Jo enjoyed Union School, and we'd hoped to start Danna there. Nova had graduated from the eighth grade just days before Connie's high school graduation and would now be going to Lakeview High. They all agreed they'd be willing to live in almost anything if they didn't have to move to town. We found a small four-room house—no indoor plumbing except for water to a sink—and not much else in the way of convenience. But it had two bunkhouses, and the children thought that sounded like an adventure. We moved into the place temporarily. In a few months we bought a home in West Side.

For Christmas that year Lynn got the family a television—our first. Bruce enjoyed it immensely, especially the educational-type programs, sports, and the Olympics. He couldn't tolerate soap operas, which pleased us. In addition he spent a great deal of time reading and helping the girls with their homework, although he continued to require long hours of rest. We felt the winter at home had been worthwhile for him. Danna, six at Christmastime, liked having Bruce around and thought it great fun to wait on her brother.

In the spring we moved into our present home. David, a tall, muscular eighteen now, joined the U.S. Navy. We dreaded his leaving. But enthusiastic and excited, he could hardly wait for the day of departure, so we just had to be happy for him. After we'd seen him off, Bruce seemed sad. He and his only brother had really been quite close.

Not long after we settled in our new home, the West Side Conservative Baptist church ceased to exist. Operating on a financial shoestring, the church had struggled for survival for some time. The cowboy preacher and his family left the community. For a while a couple of other ministers tried to keep the spiritual flames burning, but they finally faded away. It seemed a shame, for the young people's group, Bruce included, had worked so hard to construct a church building. Most of the material had been donated, and all of the labor. But because the community had lost interest, the church closed its doors.

Bruce missed his minister friend, but he didn't seem particularly eager to attend any church on a regular basis. Perhaps the embarrassment he felt with his handicap offered an excuse for staying home. Getting ready to go anywhere was a chore he'd rather avoid. He began to turn to his Bible and to radio for his spiritual needs.

The county school superintendent—a lovely, warm, unselfish person—took an exceptional interest in Bruce. Knowing that he possessed a remarkable curiosity for scientific knowledge, especially in the field of electronics and radio, she gave him a book on the subject written with the novice in mind. He read the book four times. We were pleased to see him become so engrossed in the subject, because we hadn't been too successful in arousing his interest in any hobbies. For a time he dabbled in leathercraft, but muscle spasms and lack of control of his hands prevented him from completing the intricate designs.

My husband, while at work one day, discussed Bruce's interest with Gary, one of his fellow employees.

"Why don't you suggest amateur radio to him, Lynn? It's an ideal avocation for shut-ins."

"Well, I don't know a thing about radio. I wouldn't have the vaguest idea how to go about helping him."

"Oh, that won't be any problem," Gary declared, warming to the subject. "I'm personally acquainted with a ham in Lakeview. Helping a handicapped boy would be right up his alley. Why not let me contact him and see how he feels about it?"

Lynn agreed that it seemed like a good idea. In a short while Byron Warburton, assistant postmaster in Lakeview, came to see Bruce. The rapport between the two—Bruce a teenager and Byron a middle-aged man—bordered on the uncanny. It was as if they had always known each other. Byron seemed to know just the right approach to intrigue Bruce in the hobby. In the course of one evening they had made arrangements for him to begin the complicated lessons necessary to learn amateur radio and Morse code, all required before he could obtain a license. For the next several months Bruce studied for long hours at a time. The whole learning process fascinated him. He had at last found something of interest that surpassed anything he'd ever done before.

In the meantime the muscles in Bruce's legs showed a definite increase in atrophy. Dr. Kliewer suggested we try muscular therapy for him. A qualified therapist made regular trips to Lakeview from Portland. He felt it was worth a try. The shoe corrections for his misshapen feet, ordered by an orthopedist in Klamath Falls, Oregon, after Dr. Kliewer had recommended Bruce see him, had not been any particular help. Perhaps the therapy would at least relieve the muscle spasms.

The therapist, a conscientious, efficient woman, fired with the challenge of Bruce's handicap, taught us a series of muscle exercises. They included all the muscles from the top of his head to all ten of his toes. The routine took about an hour. She expected us to do them faithfully twice a day. Bruce couldn't do them alone. It meant I would have to arrange my work schedule to include an hour each morning and afternoon to exercise him. We followed the procedure for three weeks before she returned to Lakeview. After measuring all of the muscles, she found that the ligaments back of his knees had lengthened by a few centimeters. We continued the routine for six months, but neither the muscle tenseness nor his imbalance showed any additional improvement. The exercises did seem to help him sleep better, but he began to complain of pains in his chest while performing the therapy. Until he could determine the cause of the pains, the doctor thought it best we discontinue the exercises. So one more channel of help closed for our son.

About this time the county health nurse became interested in Bruce's plight. Because of the rarity and the lack of knowledge of his ailment, his case was fast becoming a topic of interest for medically oriented persons. Bruce's balance had worsened to the extent of endangering his safety and magnifying the possibility of broken bones. He fell frequently now. Dr. Kliewer thought it best to resort to arm crutches to enable him to get about more easily and with reasonable security. The county nurse asked us to let her acquire the crutches for him through the Easter Seal Society. We were dubious about accepting the gift, for we felt we should be responsible for our son's needs just as long as we possibly could. Mrs. McKinney didn't agree.

"Do you ever contribute to the Society, Mrs. Wyman?" she asked me one day on the telephone.

"Well, yes we do, but we've never been able to afford to give a very substantial amount." Certain she would feel our yearly five or ten dollars pretty inadequate, I awaited her reply.

"It doesn't matter if you've never contributed. It's just that I thought if you had, you'd feel less like you were accepting charity. Please, I insist you let me order them for Bruce."

I relented. In a few days they arrived, and Bruce immediately took to them. We could hardly believe how much better he got about with their added security.

Only a few weeks elapsed after Bruce received the crutches when another excited call from the health nurse surprised me. She had just learned about a breakthrough on a rather complex disease not fully understood before. From the description of the symptoms, she thought it could well be what afflicted Bruce. Would I please contact Dr. Kliewer, she asked. Of course I agreed and made an early appointment with him.

He looked at the long word. "*Phenylketonuria*—Hm-m-m, well, it's a new one on me. From the word construction, I would say it pertains to the kidneys. Don't get your hopes up, but I'll find out about it just as quickly as I can."

The next day he called and asked me to bring a urine specimen from Bruce. In about a week the report came back from the laboratory—negative. His voice on the phone sounded relieved. "Thank God, Bruce doesn't have it. There'd be little hope at all for him."

The discovery of phenylketonuria seems commonplace now. Every newborn baby routinely receives a PK test before it leaves the hospital. When diagnosed at birth, medical science can control the disease with diet. Once more research had paid off—but not for Bruce.

Listening to his pocket-sized transistor radio, a cherished birthday gift, occupied much of Bruce's time. He kept up to date on every newscast and in the late afternoons listened to H. M. S. Richards' religious program. A local Adventist family, whom we knew slightly because Mr. Fullerton was a lab technician at the Lakeview hospital, sponsored the program. For many weeks my son scarcely missed a broadcast. Then for some unexplained reason, the radio station discontinued the program. Bruce was extremely disappointed.

"You know, Mom, I'd sort of like to learn more about the Adventist faith. Sounds to me like they might have something."

"Well, I suppose that could be arranged."

To begin with, he sent for a Bible study course from an address given on the radio program. He completed all the lessons, enjoying the incentive to study the Scriptures. Apparently the Voice of Prophecy organization contacted the Klamath Falls Seventh-day Adventist congregation. At that time the local church was not functional. A minister came to visit Bruce. Impressed with the man, Bruce promised to take an instruction course with the Seventh-day Adventist Church as soon as it could be arranged. Plans were in the brewing for reestablishing the Lakeview branch Adventist church.

Soon two men came and presented the course two nights weekly for Bruce. His father and I participated. After completing the lessons, Bruce seemed to need time to think the whole thing out. Lynn and I did not pursue the issue because we still held to the faith in which we'd been raised.

One of the instructors we thought a rather peculiar man, given somewhat to fanaticism. His brother often tried to reason with him. It was plain to see tension existed between the two. A few weeks after we'd completed the course, we learned that the unusual teacher had suffered a mental collapse severe enough to require that he be institutionalized. We felt sad, for he'd really been a likable fellow. But it certainly explained his unorthodox behavior. Bruce more or less lost interest. Apparently the local Adventist church stumbled along without much organization after the two men and their families left the community. No one got in touch with Bruce again. Soon we heard that the congregation had dwindled away. Bruce seemed to question the doctrine he'd learned and wondered how much of it had been factual, since the one man had been teaching under mental confusion. Still a teenager, Bruce tended to question not only religion but the validity of everything he heard or read.

Other religious broadcasts drew his attention. He began regularly to tune in Herbert W. Armstrong and the Ambassador College group. For some time their belief intrigued him. He sent for all their publications and read their periodicals from cover to cover. Not being a follower of their teachings, I engaged in some rather heated discussions with Bruce. Neither Merrie Jo nor Danna were old enough to understand much about doctrine. Nova had grown fond of a Mormon boy and had little time for Mr. Armstrong and his ideas. With his father away at work most of the time, Bruce had no one except his mother to challenge his viewpoints. With the sedentary life he was forced to lead, he needed to converse with someone. Sometimes our reasoning was more argumentative than constructive. But our deep respect for each other's opinions always won out. We'd simply change the subject.

In the meantime Bruce still worked steadily to earn his amateur radio license.

Late in the fall of 1961 Bruce suffered a bad fall. The crutches had worked well for about a year. Then their usefulness began to diminish. They frequently caught in whatever obstruction happened to be close by. This particular time Bruce braced himself with a crutch while he opened the back door with the other hand. Losing his balance, he tumbled against the door casing, one arm and one crutch outside, the other twisted under him. His legs knotted together and stiffened and tensed. I could barely pull them apart and straighten his body out on the porch floor. His face was contorted in pain. Disentangling his arms from the crutch bands, I eased him into a more comfortable position. When I pulled on his right arm, he screamed in agony. For quite a while we rested there as I bathed his sweat-laden face with a cool cloth. Inch by inch we worked our way into the living room, and I managed to lift him onto the couch. An ice pack applied to the injured arm muscles eased the pain. Bruce had no broken bones, but his arm and shoulder muscles were badly sprained. Dr. Kliewer thought it fortunate that he had not been injured seriously.

"I hate to suggest this, Dorothy and Lynn, for I realize how important it is to keep Bruce on his feet as long as we can. But it's getting too risky. One of these days it's going to be much more than sprained ligaments. You don't want that, I know."

Of course we didn't. We began to consider the best way to resort to a wheelchair. Fortunately we didn't have to wait long for an answer to our prayers. Lynn's eldest brother, George, and his wife, Dorothy, called from Los Angeles and begged us to bring the children down during Christmas vacation. They wanted to treat them to Disneyland, Knott's Berry Farm, and Marineland for a Christmas gift. The invitation seemed almost a miracle.

Coming right at Christmastime, we really couldn't afford to buy a wheelchair. They were expensive, at least the type we needed for Bruce was. Instead we rented a nice chair by the month from a medical rental service in

Klamath Falls. He loved it. It enabled him to get all about the house in absolute safety. The girls almost fought for turns to take him outside, until the novelty wore off. They soon learned how much work it took to negotiate a rough surface with a wheeled vehicle that one had to push.

Christmas Day we spent at home. The morning after found us on our way to sunny California. What a hoax! We hardly saw the sun in Los Angeles, and then only filtered through a smoke-colored sky.

Disneyland promised to be everything we'd been told it was, if we could just get through the endless lines to see it. As if Mother Nature heard the children's pleas, the weather changed in a matter of a few moments. A cool breeze blew in off the Pacific. To those warm-weather residents it felt downright chilly. The park cleared almost like magic. It didn't feel a bit uncomfortable to us eastern Oregonians, and apparently it didn't to a group of sailors just in from the northern seas. They joined us, along with a few other brave souls. Together we saw more of Disneyland in one evening than Lynn's brother and his family had seen in all the many years they'd lived in Los Angeles.

The courtesy bestowed upon Bruce and other handicapped visitors amazed us. Attendants would help us get him on a ride, even to the point of helping Lynn carry him. Then they would hurry down to the exit point and be waiting there for him with the wheelchair. Their kindness went a long way in renewing our faith in the human race.

It was a trip to remember and an excellent diversion to make the transition from crutches to a wheelchair painless for Bruce.

Chapter 6

Back from California Bruce buckled down to a rigid routine to learn the requirements for his amateur radio license. Byron worked with him hour after hour. We all began to hear dit-dit-da-da's in our sleep as Bruce played recordings of Morse code over and over and over again. An inch-thick manual in fine print and weird diagrams made absolutely no sense to me, but Bruce seemed to comprehend every word.

At Byron's suggestion we purchased a receiver for him in kit form. I couldn't imagine how we'd ever get it put together for him. My worries were needless. When it arrived, Byron and two other "ham" friends that Bruce had acquired went to work on it. In a short while they assembled the parts, and an operational radio receiver materialized out of a jumble of wires and components. All he lacked now was a transmitter, two sixty-foot poles for a dipole antenna, and rolls of something called ladder-line. Those would simply have to wait until we could afford them. The big drawback of the radio hobby—expense! Byron seemed vague about when Bruce would need them or how soon he'd be ready to take his examination. But he advised that we go ahead and order the ladder-line, since it wasn't terribly costly. We did.

Early one Saturday morning the sound of heavy equipment interrupted our breakfast. It seemed as if it would come right into the house. We rushed outside to see what could be happening. There into our driveway roared a Copco Power Company pole truck, complete with boom lift and two long lodgepole pines stripped of their limbs and ready to set. Furthermore, a crew of men were on hand to do the job. Although I shuddered to think what that would cost us, I remained quiet. Bruce beamed. In an hour or so two poles—higher than our power-line poles—sat stalwart and sturdy in the wind, connected by an antenna wire. Byron spent the afternoon attaching the ladder-line and making the necessary hookups. When my husband approached the men about paying them, wide grins spread across their faces. One who seemed to be the boss replied, "Well, you see, we don't work on Saturdays, and we couldn't charge for work we haven't done." A thank-you seemed inadequate, but the crew acted as if they'd been overpaid.

As Byron prepared to leave he shook Bruce gently by the shoulder. "I'll be out Wednesday, Bruce, just as soon as I get off work. I think you're ready for that examination." He must have been. Although nervous and tense, he completed the test without any trouble. Several weeks later the license came by mail in an impressive-looking envelope from the Federal Communications Commission. Silently Bruce fondled the little square of paper in his hands, and I saw a big tear wander down his cheek.

Only a transmitter delayed Bruce's getting on the air now. Hardly a week had elapsed after his license arrived when the sharp ringing of the telephone interrupted my dishwashing.

"Would you object if we came out to see Bruce this afternoon?" the voice almost begged. "It won't take us long." The woman seemed vague when I asked the purpose of the visit. "Well-l-l, we've a little gift for Bruce. We hoped it could be a surprise."

Still not knowing whom the voice belonged to, I told her my son enjoyed company, and I'd not mention the gift. Before I could hang up, she added, "Perhaps you wouldn't mind if we brought along a photographer?"

Good heavens, why a photographer? His room's a mess! I'll never get it cleaned before they get here. But I conceded. Bruce, never one to become unduly excited, remarked that if he could stand his room all the time, whoever was coming could surely take it for a few minutes. Not impressed with his logic, I pulled a few tricks to make a house look neat, although not really scrubbed and immaculate. While I dashed about, Bruce straightened his desk and put on a clean shirt.

An hour later, two Soroptimist Club members, accompanied by the editor of the local newspaper, presented Bruce with his longed-for transmitter.

"We work on a project every year for the benefit of the community or some Lake County resident," one of the women explained. "This year we chose Bruce to be the recipient. We couldn't think of a more worthy cause."

A Gordian knot lodged in my throat and blocked the words I wanted to say. For a moment Bruce couldn't speak either. When he tried to thank his benefactors, one of them interrupted, "You don't need any words to thank us, Bruce. That smile and the sparkle in your eyes speak loud and clear. Can you capture that look, Les?"

The editor did a fine piece of photography, complete

with the new transmitter and his receiver. Evidence of Bruce's gratefulness showed well in the following week's paper. Becoming a "ham" was a crowning achievement for Bruce.

Hours of loneliness—the frustrations of a young boy who ought to be having a social life with pretty girls and with boys his own age but couldn't—vanished. Amateur radio opened up a whole new life. Suddenly Bruce had friends around the world—dozens of them. The days lacked hours enough to fulfill all his new adventures. Life took on real purpose now.

His new friendships widened his horizons. He began to realize more fully that God's loving-kindness encompassed him. His spiritual awareness magnified, and he searched for religious truth.

Nova Lynne's interest in the Mormon religion aroused Bruce's curiosity too. Some of the members of the local stake had been friends of our family for some time. Bruce decided to take the instruction courses for their church. Various ones of their teaching missionaries conducted the classes. Intrigued, Bruce thoroughly enjoyed the sessions. But after completing them, he didn't seem eager to join their ranks. When I questioned him, he said, "There are just too many points of their doctrine I can't go along with. I won't join a church I don't agree with." It began to be more apparent as time went by that no one could persuade him to swear allegiance to anything unless he felt it was right for him. He and Nova discussed the pros and cons many times, but he never relented.

On occasion Jehovah Witnesses would stop at our door. Bruce relished Bible discussions with them—even purchased a New World Translation of the Bible from them—but that's as far as it went. More and more he read the Bible. As a hobby he began collecting various translations. He read them all. In the course of a few years—probably six or seven—he read the Bible from cover to cover eleven times.

In October, 1963, the outer edge of a freak hurricane buffeted Lake County. The damage inflicted on coastal Oregon mounted into the millions of dollars. Some areas were without normal communication. Byron Warburton called Bruce and asked if he'd be willing to stand by on the Oregon Emergency Network, an amateur radio frequency. Thrilled to be able to be of service, he never left his post for twenty-four hours. His station—K7QHM—relayed a number of messages for stranded travelers. Many western Oregon hunters, searching for the large mule deer in eastern Oregon, found themselves unable to contact relatives. For the first time in a long while Bruce felt really needed. It gave his morale a boost like nothing had that he'd ever done before. His words became a monotony. "This is King 7 Queen Henry Mary standing by. Do you copy?" Only after the emergency subsided did he relinquish his place on the air. Exhausted, he tumbled into bed and slept the clock around.

Our family decreased as the younger ones grew older. Nova Lynne decided to attend college at Brigham Young University in Provo, Utah. With David still away in the navy, only Bruce, Merrie Jo, and Danna remained at home now. The property we had purchased in West Side contained several acres but not a very large house. We obtained two bunkhouses from Weyerhaeuser Company to add on to the house and eventually create a four-bedroom home. Until we could get the work done,

Bruce and the girls occupied one of the buildings, with Bruce in a separate room. Both Merrie Jo and Danna became quite adept at shuttling Bruce in his wheelchair back and forth from the bunkhouse to the main house. At bedtime, to make it easier for Bruce, they'd sometimes work in pairs—one of them grasping him under the arms and the other his legs. Together they could quickly boost him out of the chair and into his bed. The system worked well, then later we acquired a patient-lift. With their father away at the woods camp much of the time, I could never have managed without them. They waited on him cheerfully and with such love in their hearts that, often marveling at the precious gifts God had given us, I counted my blessings many times over.

During the early winter of 1964 the chest pains that plagued Bruce when we'd practiced the muscular therapy returned with renewed vigor. We feared a heart condition, and Dr. Kliewer did an electrocardiogram. Nothing unusual showed on the graph, but still the pains persisted. He searched for a cause, and I read everything I could get my hands on that sounded like it might pertain to Bruce's case.

After reading the book *Body, Mind and Sugar* by Dr. E. M. Abramson, I learned a lot about hypoglycemia. Since diabetes ran in both Lynn's and my side of the family, I approached Dr. Kliewer with the book. Yes, he said, he was quite familiar with the blood condition, although he doubted Bruce suffered from it. But a shot in the dark was better than nothing, so he'd run a glucose tolerance test on him. Since Bruce was confined to a wheelchair, getting him to and from doctors' offices presented a problem. One of our neighbors, a registered nurse, offered to do the test in her home. Our doctor agreed and made the arrangements with her. We spent a lovely day at her house. I ironed for her while she collected the blood samples from Bruce. She wouldn't accept any other pay. People, at least almost all of them, had been so kind, so considerate, of our son. It made us truly grateful for the love others demonstrated for him.

When the result of the test returned, Bruce showed only a slight tendency toward low blood sugar. It couldn't possibly be the cause of the severe chest pain. However, the attacks continued, becoming more frequent as time progressed.

The pain was of such short duration that getting him to a doctor or the hospital during it was impossible. Dr. Kliewer suggested a nitroglycerin tablet at the onset of an attack because he felt certain it involved the heart. But the medication triggered such terrific headaches that we discontinued it. We considered a stay in the hospital so someone could run an electrocardiogram while the pain existed. But at that time bed rest eliminated the problem, and our doctor believed it a useless course. The pain being sporadic, there wasn't any certainty of its occurrence. Bruce might go for several weeks without any pain, and again he might experience the attacks two or three times a day. All we could do was to just wait for something concrete to happen.

In the meantime—part of 1963 and 1964—we took Bruce weekly to Klamath Falls for chiropractic treatments for a full year. Dr. Robert Garrison explained to us what he felt he might be able to do for him, but he warned that it might not be any more help than any other source. He worried that if he wasn't successful we perhaps would lose all faith in the art of chiropractic. But he yearned for the chance to do what he could.

"I see no reason for you to feel that way, Bob," my husband, an ardent champion of chiropractic, told him. 'We haven't lost faith in the medical profession, and we've had ample opportunity to do just that. We can't expect more of you than we've received from them. All we can do is hope."

Smiles wreathed Dr. Garrison's face. "Well then," he said, "if you can display that kind of faith in me, and Bruce can too, I have a proposition for you. I realize this is going to be an expensive as well as tiring and time-consuming venture for you. It takes a while to drive ninety-five miles here and the same back home." He warmed to the subject. "If you will take care of one treatment, I'll cover the second, and so forth."

We could hardly believe his words and said so.

"Nevertheless, that's the only way I'll do it. We're working here with a case for which I can't offer any promises. But it's a real challenge, and I'd be grateful for the chance to help if I can. After all, isn't that what doctors are for—to alleviate suffering wherever possible?"

As we thanked him and prepared to leave the office he added, "Let's keep this financial arrangement just between ourselves, OK? If Bruce knew about it, there's a remote possibility it could have a psychological effect on the treatments. I'd rather not risk it. I wouldn't want Bruce for one minute to think I was just doodling with his case."

Unfortunately chiropractic didn't bring any more cure than any other therapy Bruce had undergone. But it did lessen the muscle spasms in his legs for a while and slowed the progress of the disease. His muscles were not as tense for quite some time, and he rested better at night. So the effort was not in vain. However, the long trip finally became tiring for Bruce. Dr. Garrison, as well as Bruce, felt the treatment had reached the limit of its benefits. The chest pains occurred with every trip, and sometimes two or three times before we'd reach home. So we gave the venture up. But it had been a welcome diversion for our son. If for no other reason than that, the experiment was worth it. Bruce made one more fast friend. Often we came home a different route. There was hardly a road, mountainous or otherwise, that we didn't travel between West Side and Klamath Falls during that year. Merrie Jo and Danna usually went with us, and we all enjoyed those adventures to see what the other side of a mountain might have to offer.

In March David came home from the service. He'd been home only a week when he went to work for a lumber operation in Paisley, Oregon. It meant a forty-five mile drive twice a day. So, happy as we were to have him home, he spent little time there. In a few months he met a captivating girl, Donna, and before long they announced wedding plans.

In December, 1964, the terrible Christmas flood deluged the Northwest. Lakeview and Lake County endured its share of high water, inundated roads, bridges washed away, and livestock drowned. Whole houses floated down the Chewaucan River near Paisley. Millwork closed early because of the danger that the men would not be able to get across the river. Just as David's pickup reached solid ground, the bridge gave way and washed down the angry waters. Once again communications in the area reached a state of emergency. Bruce stood by on his ham radio as he had done the previous year. He offered assistance in relaying messages for several stranded persons. But he could not manage an around-the-clock vigil. Once again the chest pains interfered, and he had to release his duty to other willing hams.

Always a bit of a daredevil, David refused to let the high water keep him away from his bride-to-be. Bruce warned him he had received word that the Dry Creek bridge might be in danger. Since it was just a small stream, his brother saw no reason for alarm. Late that night, as he reached the center of the bridge on his way home, David felt it sway. Suddenly water engulfed him, and the headlights of his pickup wavered in and out of murky, boiling water. He gunned the motor and somehow made it across. Moments later the bridge whirled and rolled down the valley, the victim of a broken dam upstream. David returned home determined to cross no more bridges until the flood subsided. "I told you so, Buddy, but you wouldn't listen!" Bruce grinned at him.

In March David and Donna were married. Strangely, Bruce's old friend, the cowboy preacher, had returned to the community to try and reactivate the Conservative Baptist church. Since their first pastorate at West Side, his wife had passed away. The minister's heart just didn't seem to be in his work. Perhaps too many memories lingered there. Nevertheless he agreed to marry David and his fiancée. The old church, scrubbed and polished, had never looked so inviting, and it seemed to welcome the neighbors, who filled its pews. An electric organ, moved in for the occasion, provided music. A cross of artificial orchids brightened the wall above the pulpit, and flowers by the basketsful permeated the air with their fragrance. The little church was beautiful.

Bruce, tired and pale, occupied a special place in his wheelchair. Earlier in the day he had suffered a particularly intense attack of the chest pains. Connie, concern etched on her face, suggested to him, "Bruce, maybe we'd better get someone to stay with you. The wedding might be too much." For a moment he looked almost angry.

"No!"

"But it might be risky——"

"I don't care. I'm going to the wedding. If I die, I die. At least I'll see my brother married."

Bruce sat through the ceremony and the long reception afterward, and mercifully the pains came no more that day.

It was the only wedding ever held in the church. A few weeks later the doors closed again. The cowboy preacher rode away to greener pastures. The church still stands, a silent ghost of what might have been a growing spiritual center for the community.

All through the spring and early summer the chest-pain attacks increased, both in frequency and severity. Dr. Kliewer ran another electrocardiogram. Still there was no indication that the heart was impaired. Bruce's general health deteriorated, and he lost weight.

"I'm stumped. I don't know any more to do for him," Dr. Kliewer confessed as he rested his head in his hands. "But I know one thing. We're going to get him someplace where someone can find what the problem is! Would you be willing to take him to Portland again?"

We hesitated, doubtful that another trip to the clinic would reveal any more than it had in the past.

"Oh, I don't want you to take him to the clinic this time, although the university will probably be involved.

I'd like you to admit him to Good Samaritan Hospital, and we'll just leave him there until they can determine what's causing these pains. In the meantime, they might find out what he's got."

"It sounds great, Doctor." Lynn looked troubled. "But unless my company insurance will take care of most of it, there's no way we can afford it."

Kliewer smiled. "Oh, yes there is, Lynn. I know you couldn't afford this; it would cost a small fortune. But there is a special grant we can place him under. I'd like very much to do this. Would you consider it?"

"Of course, we would!" Lynn didn't bother to consult me. He grasped the opportunity as if he thought it might escape before we could take advantage of it.

"Then it's settled. I'll make the arrangements right now."

Almost a month elapsed before we could get Bruce in under the program. Late July, with its hot, muggy weather, found us on our way to Portland. Merrie Jo and Danna accompanied us. Since better than three hundred miles separate Lakeview and Portland, we planned to make a vacation excursion out of the trip and attend a wedding in Cottage Grove. One of the girls our children had played with when we lived in the old lumber camp shack had set her marriage date, and it fit right in with our schedule. But high atop Willamette Pass a violent attack of the chest pains gripped Bruce. He writhed in misery in the back seat of the stuffy station wagon, his legs jerking almost to his chin as the uncontrollable muscle spasms wracked his body. My husband pulled off into a shaded picnic area, where we made an improvised pallet on the forest floor for him. Any thought of weddings vanished as Bruce struggled to overcome the attack. We insisted he rest a couple of hours. He didn't argue, although missing the wedding disappointed him.

We made it to Cottage Grove in the evening, and Bruce rested at my nephew's most of the following day. In the afternoon he felt able to attend a dinner in Lorane given for us by our old neighbors the Suiters. Bruce enjoyed the evening and the chance to visit our friends, especially their daughter Joan, who had long corresponded with him. After a good night's rest, we traveled the remaining distance to Portland and admitted Bruce on time at the huge Good Samaritan Hospital.

Bruce had been born just across the street at Wilcox Memorial, the maternity division of Good Samaritan. Our little hometown hospital in Lakeview could well have lost itself in the reception room alone of the enormous medical facility. After a woman filled out the necessary forms for our son's admittance, a rather cute candy striper whisked us away to the sixth floor neurological department. There two orderlies, about Bruce's age, made him ready for bed and lifted him gently into white, sterile sheets. While a dark-haired registered nurse took blood samples from Bruce, a short, stocky Filipino doctor invited my husband and me into his office.

"Perhaps we can get the paper work out of the way while the routine tests are given to Bruce." He motioned us both to chairs grouped about his desk. "There'll probably be quite a lengthy history. I see Bruce has an illness of long duration."

Thus began a tedious session of trying to remember the smallest details with the help of well-worn notes. The neurologist, as had all the others, wanted complete information. When we came to the previous journeys to

Portland clinics, he held up his hand.

"Why don't we skip over this? I've been informed that Dr. Dow will be consulted sometime during Bruce's stay with us. I see no reason for you to try to remember all the medical terms they must have subjected you to. Dr. Dow's records will be available to us whenever necessary. In fact, I'd like you to understand there will be a large staff of medical persons working with Bruce."

We both sighed in relief. "This might be what we've been waiting eighteen years for!" I said.

"I sincerely hope it is, Mrs. Wyman. Are the two girls with you your son's sisters?"

"Yes, they are." *That's an unusual question*, I thought.

"That pleases me." The doctor scribbled a notation on Bruce's file. "I hope you're planning to stay in the city for a few days. We'll need to do some examinations and tests on the family too." *Well, that is a switch. We've often been questioned about his case but never examined.* My husband told him we'd planned to stay the remainder of the week.

Each day we visited Bruce. He seemed to enjoy all the attention given him, and the new routines fascinated him. While he underwent tests we took the girls sightseeing. They had their turn at the Portland zoo. Evenings with the families of my nephews made us aware of the blessings of belonging to a large and devoted family. Finally our day at the hospital laboratories arrived. We spent an entire afternoon with several staff members, who put us all through numerous nerve reaction and coordination examinations. They drew blood for analysis. The girls thought it all quite amusing and couldn't wait to tell Bruce how they were being treated.

Friday came all too soon, and we had to return to Lakeview. The doctors had hardly more than begun the work they were anxious to do with Bruce and asked that we leave him at least another week. We'd been certain before we left home it would be necessary to do this, but leaving our son alone in a strange place seemed almost too much to bear. Bruce, a little melancholy, too, didn't help the situation any. While Merrie Jo and Danna and his father joked with him, trying to make the parting easier, I walked over to the window. Across the street, blurred through my tears, stood the hospital where Bruce had first joined our family. For a moment I thought, "I can't leave him now!" But I knew that was foolish. Bruce, no longer an innocent, helpless baby, had celebrated his twenty-first birthday in April. Perfectly capable of deciding what medical procedures he would consent to, and of legal age to sign for them, I couldn't embarrass him with my apprehensions. *For once you can let him make his own decisions. Let him be the man he is!*

"Come on, Mother, we'd best be going." Lynn never called me Mother unless he felt sentimental. I peeked at Bruce. He'd already busied himself with his pocket radio. The girls had vanished into the hallway. Glancing back at the old maternity building, I tried to repress the tears that welled in my eyes. *Dear God, watch over him. Don't let him be lonely, and please give the ones who are trying to help him the wisdom they need. Father, if it's not too much to ask, bring us back safely to him.* I rushed over to him, squeezed his outstretched arm, gave him a quick kiss, and followed Lynn to the door. As I turned to wave, that waggish smile played at the corners of his mouth, and he waved back. With a prayer on my lips, I closed the door and left my son to his destiny.

The plaintive notes of the church organ seemed to hover over the baptistry and caress my son. Tony placed a folded white handkerchief over his mouth and nose and lovingly immersed him in the water. In a voice vibrant with emotion I heard him say, "Bruce, I baptize you in the name of the Father, the Son, and the Holy Spirit."

The young minister and his assistant lifted Bruce out of the pool. The swish and gurgle of the receding water broke the silence of the congregation. Suddenly the room burst with the joy of their voices.

"Yes, we'll gather at the river,
>   The beautiful, the beautiful river;
>   Gather with the saints at the river
>   That flows by the throne of God."

As Tony held Bruce, dripping and wet, on the edge of the baptistry, the resident minister raised his voice in triumphant prayer. His speech impediment vanished, and his thankful words to the Lord for the gift of a new convert rang clear and true.

With head bowed, I stole a glance at Bruce. Water coursed down his cheeks and mingled with the tears there. But his face, glowing and resplendent, mirrored the rejoicing I knew filled his heart.

The "Amen" ended the reverent silence, and Lynn stepped forward. Together he and Tony carried Bruce into an adjoining room to be dressed, and little rivulets of water left behind them a trail across the deep purple rug. I followed them out of the room.

Chapter 7

After Bruce had spent two weeks at Good Samaritan, a young man who introduced himself as Dr. James Cereghino called to say he could go home now. They had no further tests to perform. The doctor, vague about the results of Bruce's hospitalization, stated he would rather speak with us personally. We left Lakeview for Portland that evening, accompanied by David and his wife.

The heat in Portland bounced off the concrete streets and buildings. The thermometer soared to 107 degrees, an unbearable temperature in the humid area of coastal Oregon. As we entered the hospital a dark reception room and dungeonlike halls greeted us. We thought there must be a power outage but learned that they had turned off all unnecessary lighting in the hope of eliminating some of the heat. Air conditioning, serving only parts of the building normally, had succumbed to the load.

Bruce lay pale and weak in his bed, sweat oozing from every pore. He smiled as we walked into his room but demonstrated little enthusiasm at seeing us. I had never seen him look more exhausted. When we asked how he felt, he just shrugged and lay quiet. My husband, concern written on his face, grasped his hand. It hung limp in his own.

"What's the matter, fella? Is this heat too much for you?"

Bruce nodded. "Yeah, and I've had a few other problems. Doc'll tell you about them. Just make sure you talk to Jim Cereghino."

My daughter-in-law and I went in search of the doctor. When we reached the hall she placed her hand on my arm. "Mom, he looks awful! What have they done to him?"

"Well, Donna, sometimes these medical examinations can be extremely taxing on one's system. I'm sure there's an explanation. But I agree, he does look terrible."

A friendly orderly offered to locate Dr. Cereghino for us. We returned to Bruce's room. In a few moments a sandy-haired, gray-eyed young man entered and shook hands with Lynn and then each of us in turn. He laid one hand on Bruce's head.

"Well, Bruce, I'm finally getting to meet your family. They're probably wondering what we've done to you." Bruce nodded, and the doctor continued speaking. "Isn't this heat terrific? I've lived here all my life, and I've seen nothing to compare with this before!"

"Mom, Jim was born in the same hospital as me."

The doctor laughed. "Oh, you bet, Bruce and I are both good old Wilcox Memorial customers." The evident friendship between the two young men eased our concern for Bruce. Someone had cared what happened to him.

"Did you get that steak I ordered for you yet, Bruce?"

"Not yet, but the nurse said I'd get it for lunch. They'll be bringing our trays pretty soon."

"Well, I'm going to steal your folks while you eat.

You know how much we've got to talk about. See to it you eat every bite of that steak."

Dr. Cereghino suggested a cooler waiting room for David and Donna, quite aware of her obvious pregnancy, and ushered Lynn and me into a hot, stuffy office. As we seated ourselves about his desk, he shuffled through Bruce's file.

"There's no point in my trying to be indifferent. In the past two weeks I've learned a great respect for Bruce. We're good friends." He picked up a pen and doodled nervously on his desk pad. "There's no way to soften the blow. I wouldn't give you false hope." Glancing first at my husband, he then fastened his eyes on mine. "Your son is a victim of Friedreich's ataxia."

Despite the heat, I felt a chill go up my spine. The antiseptic odor of the hospital suddenly seemed overwhelming. Nauseated, I gripped the arms of my chair. Although we were not familiar with Friedreich's ataxia, the doctor's voice left no doubt in my mind. Medically speaking, our son was a hopeless invalid.

Webster's dictionary defines ataxia as an "irregularity in muscle action through failure of muscular coordination." One must delve deep into medical literature to learn that the lack of muscular coordination stems from a dysfunction of the nervous system and its complex communication with the muscles. Many diseases, some quite common, result from ataxia. Among the more familiar are chorea, multiple sclerosis, and Parkinson's disease, or the shaking palsy. In addition, a half dozen or so other ataxias have associated with them the names of the various researchers who first recognized the particular ailment. Friedreich's ataxia is one of the latter.

Since 1917 medical science has been able to diagnose the disease, discovered by Nikolaus Friedreich in 1863. However, most neuromuscular illnesses are very similar in symptoms, requiring much examination and laboratory work before the examining physician can reach a definite conclusion.

In Bruce's case an electromyogram provided the conclusive evidence. It requires the removal of a portion of muscle tissue for examination. Now, finally, a young, dedicated neurologist had tested, studied, and analyzed until, beyond reasonable doubt, he had concluded the research. The decision, of course, was not his alone, but rather that of many specialists in the field. However, in our opinion, only through the perseverance of Dr. James Cereghino had we at long last learned the name of the dread disease that crept slowly throughout Bruce's body and left him a cripple.

The doctor leaned forward, putting his elbows on the desk and covering his face with his hands. I noticed his fingernails, clean and manicured, as his fingers pressed hard on his eyelids.

"I'm sorry. I'm truly sorry. I wish——" He took his hands from his face and looked at me.

It seemed the walls of the stuffy little office would close in on me. For the first time I noticed the room had no windows. A compelling desire to see the blue of the sky, to feel a breath of fresh air, enveloped me.

Invalid—invalid—always an invalid—— The words reverberated through my mind like the throb of a migraine headache. I didn't want to look at my husband but knew that I must. He sat silent, stoic, his hands folded. But his eyes mirrored the turmoil I knew gnawed inside him. His voice broke the silence. "Are you absolutely sure?"

"As certain as we can possibly be, short of an autopsy after death." Relief flooded the doctor's face as the moment of our shock passed. He seemed glad to be back on familiar ground as he began explaining in minute detail the results of the two weeks' work with Bruce.

"I can't understand why you haven't been told long before now," he said. "True, it's a rare disease. At present there are only seventeen known cases in the Northwest." He scribbled again on the desk pad. "But it has been diagnosed quite successfully since 1917. With a case as advanced as Bruce's, it's ridiculous that someone hasn't pinpointed it before."

We could have told him why, for we'd been the long route of medical personnel too overworked to spend enough time to really study a case. Along that route we also found many others too apathetic to care, and some with too little knowledge to recognize the symptoms.

I wanted to say, "Always be as compassionate and persevering as you are, and you'll make a name for yourself in medical history." But I didn't. Instead, a torrent of questions burst forth about Bruce's welfare. Dr. Cereghino smiled. Understanding and patience showing on his countenance, he continued the long, complicated explanations.

The disease itself, he told us in simple terms, involved the death of the nerve cells in the spinal cord. As the deterioration progressed, each portion of the body served by those nerves would become impaired. Death seldom occurred from the illness itself, but rather by severe complications of it. For example, they had determined that Bruce's chest pains resulted from an enlarging of the heart and the failure of the nerves to communicate the proper impulses to the heart muscle to ensure a regular and uninterrupted heartbeat.

"He suffers agonizing pain when these attacks occur," Cereghino said. "As a matter of fact, the heart specialist (and he named a prominent one) who examined Bruce during one of the seizures and monitored the electrocardiograph marveled that they had not long since taken his life. With medication, we think we have the condition reasonably controlled."

When we inquired what treatment, medication, or cure might be possible for Friedreich's ataxia, he could only answer negatively.

"We don't even know the cause, to say nothing of a cure." Sympathy welled up in his eyes. "I can't tell you *anything* you can do for him. Actually, you've been doing for years the only things you can. Certain aspects of the disease I'm sure will help you to understand Bruce's reactions to situations." He traced the outline of a near perfect star on his desk pad. "I'll go through every detail with you. Perhaps there will be some comfort in knowing all that medical science has to offer, which isn't much."

My husband caught the doctor's eye. "Perhaps this is a little unfair to ask, but can you give us any idea of how long he will live?"

Dr. Cereghino frowned. "Well, I've never been much of a prophet. I hate to make that sort of commitment. We doctors are so often proved wrong." In silence he reassembled Bruce's file. "Many times the medical profession will say, 'You have only a year to live,' and the person ends up dying of old age. Again we say, 'You've many years ahead of you,' and the patient may go out the next day and get killed in an accident or have a heart attack. But I would say, with the speed of progression

Bruce is experiencing now, optimistically ten years."

Somehow, down through the years, we'd clung to the hope that if someone could properly diagnose his illness, there might be a cure—if not healing, then at least therapeutical rehabilitation. But just nothing—it was too much to accept. I couldn't believe the finality of it all. But God still remained omnipotent and present. If one He created lived, there must yet be hope!

The young physician followed us back to Bruce's room. As we walked slowly down the darkened halls he said, "I'd like you to know how well adjusted and intellectually phenomenal we think Bruce is for a handicapped person. I feel privileged to know him. He's been a real inspiration to me and a number of others in this neurological department."

We thanked him, and I felt proud to know that our son, though disabled, fulfilled a real purpose in life. How fortunate we were to have been chosen to be his parents.

As we neared his room Lynn, always one to look forward instead of back, asked the doctor, "What's this about a steak for Bruce's lunch? Isn't that fare a little unusual for a hospital?"

Dr. Cereghino laughed. "It is at that. Well, you see, Bruce couldn't tolerate synthetic digitalis. We had to go to the natural whole leaf. Until the synthetic drug got out of his system, he lost every meal. Some know-it-all dietitian decided he should have a liquid diet. It didn't appear on his charts, and Bruce didn't tell me until this morning." He looked perturbed. "Such a diet he doesn't need! So I ordered a steak." He chuckled. "There are a few ears burning in the nutrition department!"

We had traveled only a few miles into the mountains

on our way home when the air blew cool and refreshing into the muggy, hot station wagon. Snow-capped Mt. Hood loomed above us. But it was apparent that Bruce, too exhausted to make the trip home that day, would have to rest. We rented a rustic log cabin, actually a three-bedroom motel-house, near the little roadside town of Rhododendron, Oregon. A gurgling stream rolled and tumbled down its rocky bed to the valley below. The tranquil music of its passing lulled Bruce into a sound sleep. The next morning he awoke refreshed and eager to be on the way again. His response, as we reached the dry, high desert area beyond Mt. Hood, amazed us. Contrary to the usual patient with a heart condition, Bruce felt much better in a high altitude. The trip to West Side continued without any further stops except for meals.

For several days Bruce spent long hours in bed resting and discussing, whenever he felt inclined, the experiences he'd had at Good Samaritan. He didn't dwell on the finality of his handicap. I could not help but wonder how shattering the diagnosis of his disease had been to his hope. As if sensing my anxiety, he said one day as we read the Bible together, "Mom, I've known for a long time that if I am ever a well person it will only be through the power of God." He made the statement calmly, no bitterness in his voice. I breathed a prayer of thankfulness for a son who was able to accept his destiny without railing against God or anyone else.

In the middle of August Nova married her Mormon sweetheart, Tom. Bruce, unable to make the journey to Ontario, Oregon, for the ceremony, remained at home under the care of David and his wife. Donna, a sympathetic, understanding girl, always went out of her way to offer her assistance in Bruce's care. We became as close as if she'd been my own daughter.

Merrie Jo and Danna were excited about the prospects of a new brother-in-law. Bruce had gone to school with Tom, and they'd had great times together as fellow Boy Scouts. It was hard to leave Bruce at home, because we knew how much the marriage meant to him. Being left out of so many things seemed an especially cruel part of his affliction. But at the same time, with a large family, Lynn and I had to be careful not to neglect our unhandicapped children. So we left him, as we had before and have many times since, resolving to enjoy ourselves for the sake of our other children and our own sanity.

The ceremony was a beautiful and altogether happy occasion. We took pictures for Bruce and brought back a piece of the wedding cake to help him capture the joyfulness of the moment.

Life has a way of skipping along—or limping, as the case may be—one day after the other, like climbing a ladder rung by rung. No matter how shattered the hopes of one day, one always has another to rebuild on. We tried to live each day to its fullest, counting our blessings and accepting the challenges of making the most out of the situations presented to us. As a family, we were fast learning that it was not the smooth road that developed one's skill, but rather the one riddled with ruts, strewn with boulders, and full of narrow places bordering the edge of the precipice. Yet as long as we allowed God to do the steering, we could be assured of safe passage. Nothing had really changed, and we all, including Bruce, found that life was good.

Bruce had acquired nieces and nephews—five of

them now. Each one vied for his attention and waited for a chance to catch him out of his wheelchair, a fascinating piece of machinery for exploring hands. They loved to maneuver it about the house. The babies thought it a special treat when he gave them a ride on his lap. Without realizing it, they learned to accept the fact that all people are not exactly alike. It developed a tolerance in them for others and a compassion that has grown with them as they mature.

With Merrie Jo and Danna in their teens and involved in various school and community projects, it was a good thing that we had completed the major remodeling of our home. It provided Bruce a room where he could spend all the time he wished at his radio in warm comfort.

Again the local radio station, KQIK, aired the "Voice of Prophecy" with H. M. S. Richards. Bruce still listened to the Ambassador College group, but now he had the opportunity to compare their faiths. More and more he shuttled his time into religious channels and began to indicate a desire to be baptized. He spent long hours reading the Bible and other inspirational books, periodicals, and whatever he could get his hands on. In fact, he studied the Scriptures with such intensity that we became uneasy about the situation. From childhood Bruce had been inclined to overdo anything that captured his interest. In our opinion, God's Biblical directive to be temperate in all things applied to all phases of life, religion included—not to neglect spirituality but to make certain the human mind is given a well-rounded mental diet to ensure its proper function. Bruce had interests in many things—tuna-fish sandwiches, science fiction, electronics, radio, politics, religion—and would bury himself in one or the other of them to the exclusion of everything else. It taxed the imagination of the entire family to steer his intellect and extensive free time into a variety of directions. It wasn't always accomplished smoothly and without contention.

During her junior and senior years of high school, Merrie Jo struck up a friendship with a neighbor boy that grew, as the months rolled by, into a lasting love affair. Bruce delighted in teasing her about her buddy that so soon became her fiancé. In November, 1966, she and Bob were married. Once again Bruce had to forgo the wedding ceremony as the young couple chose to go to Reno, Nevada, to pledge their vows. But we returned the 257 miles to Lakeview immediately after the ceremony. Bruce attended, along with many friends and neighbors, the reception David and Donna gave the young couple. Although he could not go out into the stormy night to assist the young people in decorating the car, Bruce made certain each one had plenty of material to get the job done.

With Merrie Jo living in Ashland, where her husband attended Southern Oregon College, Bruce missed her pleasant disposition. She and Bob came home as often as they could, but even so, he and Danna went through a period of loneliness. As a result, they turned to each other and became closer than ever.

When Danna came home from school in the evening, Bruce eagerly awaited the account of not only her day's activities but those of her friends and classmates as well. He often helped Danna with her homework, or if time permitted, they'd just chat. Danna loved the out-of-doors, and her projects consumed most of the daylight hours in the evening. She raised rabbits and sheep and always helped me with the main sheep flock, especially during lambing season, when she was my right hand. We always had an old ewe who refused to accept her new baby. My daughter would take the lamb to the house if the mother had let it become chilled, which happened often. With the oven door open for heat, she and Bruce would nurse the tiny ball of wool back to life. When the weather permitted, she'd roll Bruce in his wheelchair to someplace where he could watch the chores being done. He particularly enjoyed the gamboling of the lambs as they played.

One day, when I had finished my outside work and returned to the house, I found Bruce intent on watching a pair of lambs in a box. One of them clung tenaciously to life, which was a bit unusual. They generally give up easily. It had lived longer than I'd expected. When I asked Bruce if he thought the lamb would make it, he replied, "Well, I think she's got a good chance. I've been praying for her."

"Praying?"

"Well, why not? If God watches over the sparrows, I'm sure He'd do the same for a little lamb. After all, they are all His creatures. We think nothing of praying for people, why not animals?"

I couldn't argue with that type of logic, so I sent my prayer along too. The lamb lived to become one of the best mothers in our herd.

In 1967 Bob and Merrie Jo had a beautiful baby boy. Little Bradley made our seventh grandchild, and I went to Ashland to assist with the new baby. Bruce had long wanted to visit his sister Connie and her family in Crescent City, California. Bradley's arrival made a golden opportunity to do just that.

I stayed only a week at my daughter and son-in-law's, but Bruce elected—at Connie's insistence—to remain in Crescent City for five or six weeks. It was the longest period he had ever been away from home. The experience relaxed him and removed a lot of the monotony that had crept into his life. He needed a change of pace from the daily routine at home.

Although routine is a necessary part of a shut-in's life, it is not a panacea. The family of the handicapped, or those responsible for their well-being, must constantly remember the necessity for change, if nothing more than a few hours away from the unvaried habits.

While Bruce enjoyed the invigorating Pacific breezes, Danna and I planned a homecoming surprise. We redecorated his room. After painting the walls, we laid a new rug, hung pretty curtains, and refinished his furniture. On the day of his arrival, Danna bubbled over with excitement. As the brother-in-law carried Bruce into the house Danna insisted he close his eyes, not allowing him to open them until she gave the word. When Clyde had laid him gently on his bed, she said, "OK, Bruce!"

For a moment a blank expression enveloped his face. Then as he realized the difference in his once-rather-drab room, that whimsical smile played across his features. Danna, bursting with pride, anxiously awaited his reaction.

"Well, how do you like it?"

"I thought something sure smelled funny in here!" he replied. With that remark Danna landed in the middle of him, and they engaged in a mild scuffling match, their equivalent of "Welcome home, Bruce!" and "I'm glad to be back, Sis!"

Early in 1968 my husband and I had to make a distant journey to attend a funeral. Merrie Jo offered to come home and care for her brother. We hesitated to leave him. For some time he'd been engrossed in spiritual awareness and various other deep subjects. Attempts to channel his thoughts into lighter areas had failed. He insisted on periods of fasting, which his crippled body could not tolerate. His appetite, never good, had so lessened that getting him to eat enough had become a real problem. Thinking perhaps Merrie Jo's arrival would accomplish the change we'd been hoping for, we left him in her care.

We were only gone four days, but when we returned, Merrie Jo was almost sick from worry about him. All her efforts to improve his condition had failed. His color ashen and his eyes sunken and lackluster, he had rapidly lost weight. Always so mentally alert, his confused reasoning frightened us. His extensive knowledge of the Bible, the sciences—especially electronics and radio—and his interest in politics had become so mingled in his mind that he could no longer differentiate between them. Although he recognized family and friends, he seemed skeptical of their relationship toward him. He distrusted those whom he loved the most. Bruce suffered hallucinations and succumbed to outbursts of laughter, tears, or anger for no apparent reason.

His condition continued for many weeks, with periodic transformation into normality that defied explanation. At times his health would slip so low that life seemed barely a flicker. A half hour later he'd be singing at the top of his voice, clamoring for something to eat, and ready to be up and about. The change might last a week or less than a day. Sleep eluded him, and he often went for thirty-six to forty-eight hours without proper rest. Sometimes he refused to eat or take his medication. Frequently only Danna, or one of the nieces or nephews, could persuade him to cooperate. The frightening situation so exhausted me that I began to fear for my own sanity. Finally, in April, Dr. Kliewer insisted we hospitalize him.

The doctor called in a local heart specialist to assist him, and together they ran more electrocardiograms. They took additional X rays and found that his heart had enlarged noticeably since the last examinations. The specialist determined that his heart, due to nerve impairment, was not utilizing the oxygen from the bloodstream. As a result, his brain cells experienced oxygen depletion, which in turn prevented proper mental functioning. The condition could vary rapidly, depending upon the nerve impulses to the heart. It was the first time Friedreich's ataxia had affected his mind. Such behavior occurs as an unusual quirk of the disease.

Bruce remained in the hospital only a few days. The only way anyone could seem to help him was to adjust his medication. We took him home, determined to do the best we could for him, though both doctors warned us that the problem could be permanent.

April slipped into May, and still Bruce showed little improvement. Our families, of many different faiths, but all deeply religious, became quite concerned about the situation. Bruce's brother and sisters, with the exception of Danna, all lived great distances from him. But each cared and was gravely anxious for his welfare.

"Thou art the God that doest wonders: thou hast declared thy strength among the people," Psalm 77:14 tells us. Again, Psalm 96:3 urges us to "declare his wonders among all people." Without consulting each other, five of Bruce's relatives—his sister Nova, a Mormon; Connie, a member of the Assembly of God; my sister Gladys, a Catholic; and my brother Earl and sister Hazel, Nazarenes—all requested special prayer services for him in their various churches on the exact same day. Each had so informed us the day afterward. But they really didn't need to tell us. We were certain our own prayers had been answered, for Bruce showed definite signs of improvement. It was a miracle. Neither Bruce nor any of our large family ever doubted its origin.

His progress continued. By the time summer arrived, he could enjoy the out-of-doors as well as he had for many summers. The anguish of his illness vanished and his disorientation disappeared. However, he never regained the phenomenal capacity for knowledge he once possessed. The drive he'd always displayed was gone. His mental faculties were still intact, but he no longer seemed to have the energy to pursue the subjects that once intrigued him. He abandoned his radio except for occasional bursts of interest. His Bible remained the one thing to which he clung. With a sort of desperation he searched the Scriptures. Although he didn't fear death, he wanted to be sure he had made all the commitments considered necessary. And he still longed for a church home.

During his illness he asked me to contact for special prayer one of the radio churches in which he'd been interested. I did. The only response he received was some brochures expounding the evils of spirit possession and a warning that unless he cast them off he could expect his mental confusion to continue. I never heard him listen to that group again.

An anointing and prayer by a bishop of the Mormon Church, at Nova's request, left him humble and gratified. But being so confused mentally at the time, he could scarcely remember his coming.

The "Voice of Prophecy" and H. M. S. Richards became a steady part of his routine now. Seldom missing a broadcast, he sent for a number of their publications and read again, when he felt up to it, the writings of Ellen G. White. He spoke often of his desire for baptism. But when we suggested arranging for the minister of the First Baptist Church, one of his good friends, to perform the service, Bruce declined.

It tired him to read for long periods now. When he requested it, I read to him while I fed him his meals. The local Grange had donated a hospital bed for his use. It made him much more comfortable and enabled us to care for him with less difficulty on our part. If he didn't feel like getting up, he could recline while I fed him, and we could enjoy a good book together. The bed, rather an antique, operated manually, but Bruce enjoyed it.

The years passed one by one. After diagnosing Bruce's handicap, Dr. Cereghino had warned us that the disease alternated between good and bad health. This became more apparent after his extreme illness in 1968. He went from periods of being quite well to times of exhaustion, heart reactions, and general physical deterioration. We were fortunate that he seldom suffered from the colds, influenzas, or viruses common to most everyone else. On occasion the oxygen problem would return, but only in mild form. For the most part he remained in full control of his mental capacities.

In 1971 Danna married a boyfriend of long standing. She and Steve said their vows in the Church of Christ in

Lakeview. Bruce attended the wedding and participated in the fun-making from his wheelchair. By now he had acquired eleven nieces and nephews, and our family made a sizable group to assemble for pictures during the reception. It was a happy occasion, although I'm sure Bruce disliked having his sister leave home. But she and her husband lived close and came often to see him. Steve, a baseball fan, spent hours talking with Bruce about their favorite sport. For many years Bruce had followed the various ball clubs and never missed a game of the World Series. He thoroughly relished a brother-in-law that was willing to discuss the plays with him.

April, 1973, heralded Bruce's twenty-eighth birthday. David and his wife and some of their close friends decided to give a dinner and dance in his honor. They rented the Grange hall, and a local band offered to play for free. More than one hundred friends and neighbors gathered to help him celebrate. In lieu of gifts, the guests and family members donated funds toward an electric bed for him. Since he was bedfast much of the time now, they realized how pleasant it would be for him to lie or sit at his own convenience. Also I'm sure they knew how many steps it would save his family. I doubt that any of them imagined how successful their venture would be, for an electric bed, even at that time, cost nearly five hundred dollars. Donations came from as far away as Seattle, Washington; Denver, Colorado; and Fond du Lac, Wisconsin. When we tallied them up, the fund contained almost four hundred dollars.

As the family sat about a warm fire after the party, marveling over the goodness of our friends and neighbors, Steve became serious. He drew his chair close to Bruce.

"Bruce, you know that I just received an insurance trust left to me by my dad before he died. I'm sure he'd have wanted me to do something worthwhile with it, and I think he'd have liked to have a part in your birthday celebration." He pulled his wallet out, carefully counted out five twenty-dollar bills, and laid them in Bruce's lap. "Danna and I want you to have your electric bed right now."

We purchased the bed and had it assembled in his room as soon as Montgomery Ward & Co. could ship it to Lakeview. Lynn and I added an adjustable hospital-type table. Bruce especially appreciated the fact that he could adjust his posture without having to wait for his mother or someone else to make him comfortable.

Just a few days after his birthday a member of the Beta Sigma Phi sorority called to ask how much more we needed for his bed. When I informed her we had already ordered it she sounded disappointed.

"Well, it looks like we blew that one. We thought we'd like to help. Those West Siders are certainly there when they're needed, aren't they?" I agreed and added that we thought they were among the finest people in the world.

"I'm sure they must be. I've heard that so many times," she said. "Well, there'll surely be another opportunity." I tried to convey my sincere appreciation to her, and we ended the conversation.

Little more than a week later the editor of the local weekly telephoned to ask if Bruce would be available for pictures in his new bed. He'd like to do a human-interest story.

"Since we've already done a couple of articles on Bruce, I think the readers would be interested in another one." I couldn't refuse his kind gesture, and we set a time for the photographs. In addition to the story about his radio transmitter years before, David's small daughter, Trina, in a conversation with Santa Claus, had asked if he wouldn't please give her Uncle Bruce something to help him walk. Santa had contacted the editor. The story, complete with a picture of her on Santa's lap, made the front page.

When Les Shaw arrived, he didn't come alone. With him was the woman from the Beta Sigma Phi group and the owner of an appliance and furniture shop in Lakeview. Between them they carried a sixteen-inch color television. It hadn't taken the sorority long to find another way to be kind to our son. To assist them, Mr. Seibert had given them the set at cost and fashioned a remote control for it at his own expense to simplify its operation for Bruce. Too choked to speak, Bruce could only smile his gratitude. Once again Les captured it on film. And too tearful for words, I could only bow my head in a moment of silent prayer for the kindness and compassion of our friends—the wonderful people in Lake County, Oregon.

My husband and Tony laid Bruce gently on a pallet on the floor of the tiny church office. The young minister excused himself, and Lynn helped me remove his saturated clothing. Bruce engaged in some small talk but refrained from any comment on the spiritual significance of his baptism. Obviously it had been a magnificent personal experience for him, one that he'd rather not diminish with explanations even to his parents. He seemed eager to get back to the service. We hurriedly toweled and dressed him, then lifted him into his wheelchair. With a final quick brush at the wrinkles in his clean pants, I stepped aside and opened the door. Lynn wheeled him into the sanctuary.

Chapter 8

The sunbeams shining through the violet-hued cross in the stained-glass window above the baptistry blended into the deep purple carpeting and danced off the azaleas that sat on the pulpit. Each face in the congregation reflected the joy that pervaded the room. One could feel the presence of the Saviour.

The wheelchair in which Bruce sat could not imprison the exaltation bursting from his heart and mirrored on his face. He had found his church home, and the pride he felt for his new spiritual family welled deep in his dark eyes. The long, long search had ended.

The organist played the opening chords of a final hymn. As the congregation rose to their feet their voices broke into such praise the entire church seemed to vibrate with their jubilation. The song of devotion concluded, and the minister offered the benediction, asking God's special blessing upon their new member. He had scarcely finished his Amen when the congregation gathered about Bruce to wish him well and welcome him into their midst.

As soon as Tony had shaken his hand in greeting, he came to me and my husband. "Bruce is really happy, don't you think?" Tony understood the extended search he had made for just the right faith. Perhaps he felt a little uneasiness for Bruce—a twinge of doubt as to whether he would be satisfied. I took his hand in mine.

"Tony, if you could have seen the determination in him when he refused to associate himself with any other church, you would know, without any skepticism, that Bruce is supremely happy. We'll always be grateful to you for your part in helping him to decide."

He started to speak but instead lowered his head and pressed my hand. Without another word he strode toward the dining room where a potluck dinner waited. I looked at Lynn. His eyes, misty with tears, followed the student minister out of the sanctuary. For a fleeting moment his arm held me tight.

"You go ahead and help with the dinner," he said. "I'll get Bruce." As I pursued Tony toward the kitchen and dining area I remembered how easily his friendship with Bruce had developed.

During the fall and winter of 1972-73 a neighbor couple became interested in Pastor George Vandeman's "It Is Written" broadcast on television. After enrolling in the Bible study course, they were surprised to have one of the church members from Klamath Falls contact them at their home to offer his assistance with the lessons. In the course of the conversation one day, he asked Bud and Shirley if they knew anyone else in the West Side area that might be interested in Bible study. Knowing Bruce's religious preferences, they suggested that perhaps he would like to speak with him, especially since he was a shut-in. Thus it was that Tony Finch came to see our son.

The two young men seemed to possess a certain rapport—a rather unusual understanding and respect for each other. Over the weeks their acquaintance blossomed into a steadfast friendship. Tony did not insist that he agree with him on every issue. Neither did he ridicule any other faith, which meant a lot to Bruce. Their conversations were not always religiously oriented. They enjoyed discussing a wide range of topics. Being young men, with only a few years between them, they had much in common.

When Bruce told us he had prayed much about the matter and had come to the conclusion that he wanted to join the Seventh-day Adventist Church, we were not surprised. So this Sabbath day in April, 1973, he had taken the final step. We were overjoyed for him, and at the same time we felt a sense of relief that he could at last have peace.

For several weeks Bruce reveled in the glory of his chosen religion. He became absorbed in the activities of the church. Through the kindness of a young family, who had recently joined the church, too, Bruce attended services nearly every Sabbath. He accepted a position on a committee and felt proud to have the group meet in his home. It pleased us to see him so engrossed in the projects and completely at ease in his own element. But he tired quickly and in a short time began showing signs of exhaustion.

In July we hosted a family reunion at our home in the country. Bruce, excited and eager for the affair to be a complete success, could hardly wait for the relatives' arrival. Family ties seemed to mean a great deal more to him than most young men his age. Perhaps some of it stemmed from the fact that he had more time to ponder the need for love in a family group. Whatever the reason, he determined to make the most of the gathering.

Some of the members came from distant states, and

because of the long distances, we had arranged to have the reunion extend over a week. Before the last guests departed, we were aware that Bruce showed signs of the heart-oxygen problem. But because we realized how much the association with his cousins, aunts, and uncles meant to him and how happy the presence of his brothers, sisters, nieces, and nephews made him, we elected to let him enjoy himself for as long as possible. Bruce had always felt that to forgo all pleasure, so that he might live a little longer, wasn't always expedient. We were inclined to agree with him. So we did not cancel the reunion or cut it short. We made him as comfortable as we could, gave him every opportunity for rest, and let him relish the things he wanted to do. When it was over he spent a week in bed.

For a few weeks he showed improvement, but as the heat of the summer increased, his physical condition worsened. He tried desperately to keep up with his church commitments, but his worn body could not stand the additional strain. He lapsed into a series of heart attacks that dwarfed any previous reaction. His heartbeat developed a break in rhythm. The two valves beat separately, one faster than the other. It became so serious Dr. Kliewer and his new partner, Dr. Robert Bomengen, entered him in Lake District Hospital for cardioversion.

They scheduled it for early Monday morning. Sunday afternoon we took him to the hospital. Several members of his church asked permission to come to the hospital for a prayer service in Bruce's behalf. In the absence of the local minister, a group from the Klamath Falls congregation also flew to Lakeview to assist the local elders.

I shall never forget how the setting sun brightened the intensive care unit of the hospital that evening. As the men gathered about Bruce and extended their prayers heavenward the sun broke through the threatening thunderheads and beamed across Bruce's bed. Everyone in the room seemed suddenly to sense that the prayers had been heard. Bruce's features relaxed. Brave though he had always been when faced with a physical problem, he had feared the cardioversion. Later, when the doctor made his evening rounds, he found that Bruce's condition had improved. By Monday morning the two valves were beating simultaneously. The doctors canceled the cardioversion.

Although he was bedfast most of the time, for three weeks Bruce's health rallied. Then, almost overnight, he slipped into a frightening relapse. A state of mental confusion gripped him that left him in anguish and exhausted his family and those who cared for him. Despite four medications, he continued to decline. We struggled with the situation at home until we saw no alternative except to hospitalize him again.

For some unknown reason the mentally disoriented often turn on those they've trusted the most. They see them as enemies and develop a fear of them that is too pathetic to describe.

Bruce was no exception. He became so frightened of me that he refused to eat or drink anything I offered him. He actually believed I was trying to kill him or that I was some harmful creature who only looked like his mother. Although I understood the psychotic reaction, it broke my heart. Even from the security of his hospital bed he stared at me with terror in his eyes. Although he mistrusted all his family, he didn't fear them as he did me.

Both Dr. Kliewer and Dr. Bomengen tried to console me with the knowledge that his reaction was not uncommon. I appreciated their concern, but I could only pray that the condition would not last.

The doctors' prognosis left us discouraged. Unable to see little indication that he would recover, they recommended we place him in a nursing facility on a permanent basis.

I flatly refused. This was my son, and I would care for him as long as I had a breath left in my body. But deep within I knew I could no longer handle the situation—he required far more care than I could give. My husband, well aware that I had reached the end of my strength, agreed with the physicians. But mother love was slow to give up.

Finally Dr. Bomengen said to me, "Dorothy, let's put it this way. We don't have to put Bruce in the nursing home, but if we don't, in a short while we'll have to put you there. Where will that leave Bruce?" I thought he exaggerated the predicament, but I couldn't argue with his logic.

Lynn drove home slowly that evening. In his calm, steady manner he convinced me that for Bruce's sake we had to give him the best care available. "I think you don't realize how worn out you really are. At least let's give this a try."

Both of us, reluctant to remove him from the security of his home, nevertheless had to make a decision. It was the most heartbreaking thing we'd ever done. With common sense the victor, we placed Bruce in the Lake District Nursing Facility in November, 1973. At the time, his mind was so impaired it made little difference to him. The nursing home occupied one wing of the hospital, and it seemed as if he'd only been moved from one room to another.

I could scarcely believe the collapse of my own energy when the responsibility for his care shifted to others. A fatigue I had never before experienced engulfed me until I could have slept for a month. But at the same time, I slept so fitfully that for about six months I would hear Bruce calling in the night. I'd find myself in his room with the light turned on before I awoke enough to realize I'd been dreaming. Then I began to appreciate the truth of the doctor's admonition and to understand what a selfish attitude I'd had toward my son. With such weariness, I couldn't possibly have given Bruce the constant care he needed. Mother love, like that of young romance, is often blind.

The staff at the nursing home, especially the attractive, black-haired, diminutive Irish supervisor, had one thought in mind—make their charges happy, give them the best care possible, and do it with a lot of tender, loving care. In no time at all Anne Murphy had gained Bruce's confidence. With the doctors' constant vigil, they soon pinpointed a number of things to work on. They found a low potassium level, discontinued some of the medication that seemed to aggravate the mental condition, and monitored his reactions to the most trivial circumstances. After a few months he gained weight and recaptured most of his mental faculties. Although he often begged to come home, when he did he would sigh in relief on returning to his familiar quarters. After the spaciousness of the nursing home, our house seemed to give him a sort of claustrophobia. If our grandchildren were about, their chatter irritated him, although he loved them dearly. Sometimes, if his physical condition was good, he would enjoy a day or a weekend at home. But generally speaking, he was never quite as content there as he thought he would be.

Several years have slipped past since Bruce began his new life. He is not always well, but the heart reactions have almost vanished. In other areas the Friedreich's ataxia has taken its toll.

Christmas of 1974 was an especially depressing time for him. Danna's husband, Steve, met death in a tragic accident six days before the holiday. Bruce received the news calmly, but tears coursed down his cheeks. "Why," he asked of no one in particular, "did it have to be Steve? Why not me? I'm so useless!" One of the rare times he ever questioned God's divine omnipotence, it was merely the result of shock. Now, he has a new brother-in-law and a lovely step-niece. Bruce cherishes Mike and Sandi just as he does all his family.

His new home has many advantages. He has many more friends to know, participates in planned activities, and attends numerous church services, if he wishes, in his own faith and many others. Recently a sympathetic physical therapist has interested him in a new electrical concept of typing for the handicapped. The possibilities excite him. He is even contemplating a sermon he hopes someone in his church will relay to the congregation. Periodically he still visits us at home and celebrates birthdays and holidays, or even just a weekend, here when he is well and the weather permits.

In recent years medical science has had some success with its research in Friedreich's ataxia. It is the general opinion now that recessive genes transmitted by the parents cause it. If Lynn and I had each married someone else, there would not be a handicapped Bruce. But then there wouldn't be a Bruce, would there? In most families where the disease appears it afflicts more than one child. In our family of seven it struck only one. I believe that if the cause is genetic, there must surely have to be other contributing factors.

A National Friedreich's Ataxia Foundation has formed. Also the Friedreich's Ataxia Group in America, Inc., with headquarters in Oakland, California, is an active organization, to which Bruce belongs. Recently the Muscular Dystrophy Foundation included FA victims in their group. Things are looking up for the sufferers of this disease.

Bruce is happy. Although his eyesight has failed and his speech is unintelligible, both debilitating consequences of Friedreich's ataxia, he still greets us with that captivating smile. He can no longer feed himself or even grasp a friend's hand in a hearty handshake. His Bible lays untouched, for he can neither see to read it nor has he the strength to hold it. Now he listens to tapes of the Scriptures from "The Voice of Prophecy." Tears of love still flow when he hears God's word of promise and good tidings—*"Verily, verily, I say unto you, he that heareth my word, and believeth on him that sent me, hath everlasting life"* (John 5:24).

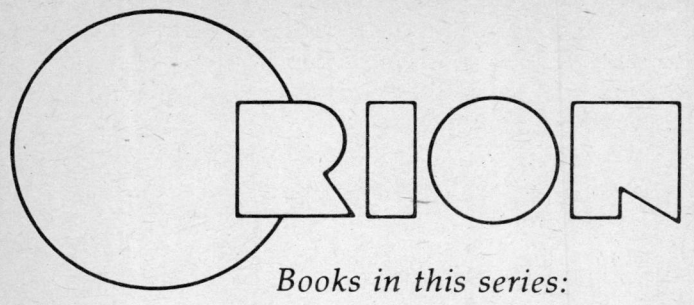

Books in this series:

Jonie Goes to Academy
Jonie Graduates
The Compleat Parent
The Compleat Marriage
Bruce
Flee the Captor
A Mink's Story
Unblessed
Where Are We Running?
Witnesses Through Trial

To my very dear
young friend.
 Love
  Elaine